ATLAS OF
MEDICAL HELMINTHOLOGY
AND
PROTOZOOLOGY

CHURCHILL LIVINGSTONE
Medical Division of Longman Group UK Limited

Distributed in the United States of America by Churchill Livingstone Inc., 1560 Broadway, New York, N. Y. 10036 and by associated companies, branches and representatives throughout the world.

First Edition	1966
Second Edition	1975
Reprinted	1976
Reprinted	1979
Reprinted	1981
Reprinted	1982
Reprinted	1984
Reprinted	1985
Reprinted	1987

ISBN 0-443-01222-9

Library of Congress Catalog Card Number
74-81190

Produced by Longman Group (FE) Ltd
Printed in Hong Kong

ATLAS OF
MEDICAL HELMINTHOLOGY
AND
PROTOZOOLOGY

BY

H. C. JEFFREY
C.B.E., M.D., F.R.C.P.E., F.R.C.Path., D.T.M. & H.

Major-General (Retd.), National Medical Director, Scottish National
Blood Transfusion Service. Formerly Director of Army Pathology and
Consulting Pathologist to the Army

AND

R. M. LEACH, B.E.M.
The Royal Army Medical College, London

SECOND EDITION

CHURCHILL LIVINGSTONE
EDINBURGH LONDON AND NEW YORK
1975

TO
ANNA and IONA

PREFACE TO THE SECOND EDITION

It is with great regret that I record the death of my collaborator in the first edition of this Atlas, Robert Leach, in 1967.

I would like to express my thanks and appreciation to the reviewers of the first edition; most of their constructive comments have been incorporated in this edition.

There have been advances in the understanding of the status of some of the protozoa, particularly of *Toxoplasma gondii* and the sarcosporidia, but until this work is finalised, alteration to the relevant parts of the Atlas is considered premature.

The new cover has been designed to emphasise the world-wide distribution of helminthic and protozoal infections, and hence the importance of all medical men having a knowledge of them.

HUGH C. JEFFREY.

Edinburgh, 1974.

PREFACE TO THE FIRST EDITION

With modern high-speed travel and population movements, doctors anywhere may be called upon to attend patients suffering from helminthic or protozoal disease ; a knowledge of the parasites causing these is becoming more and more a necessity for all medical men.

This Atlas has been designed primarily as a visual aid to teaching, with the object of illustrating systematically the life-cycles and main morphological features of the worms and protozoa affecting man, with a minimum of text.

It has been divided into three Parts. The first two, dealing with the commoner worms and the protozoa, are designed for students and post-graduate refresher courses. The third part, dealing with the parasitic worms in more detail, is designed for candidates for the Diploma in Tropical Medicine and Hygiene and for those actually working in the areas where these parasites are found.

There is necessarily some overlap between Parts I and III, but this is deliberate. Recapitulation is a necessary part of teaching and it is hoped that the simpler handling of Part I will make Part III easier to understand, and to learn, when the time comes for the post-graduate student to study these parasites in more detail.

As knowledge of the pathological processes in any disease is the foundation for an understanding of the clinical manifestations, attention has been paid to clinico-pathological correlation, this being dealt with particularly in Plates 42, 59, 62 and 64 for protozoal infections, and in Plates 114-121 for infections with worms.

A number of the illustrations have been re-drawn from material previously prepared for MacFarlane's Short Synopsis of Human Protozoology and Helminthology, 1960 and we are most grateful to Brigadier L. R. S. MacFarlane, C.B.E., and our publishers for permission to use these. The remainder are original and prepared for this Atlas.

Finally we are most indebted to various members of the staff of the Royal Army Medical College, London, for constructive criticism of the plates as they were designed.

HUGH C. JEFFREY.
ROBERT M. LEACH.

Singapore and London, 1966.

PART I

The commoner worms of medical importance.

CONTENTS

PLATE

Initial classification of worms of medical importance   1

Nematobe worms

      Ascaris lumbricoides   2

      Trichuris trichiura   3

      Enterobius vermicularis   4

      Strongyloides stercoralis   5

      Ancylostoma duodenale   6

      Necator americanus   6

      Trichinella spiralis   7

            Pathology of trichiniasis   8

      Wuchereria bancrofti   9

      Brugia malayi   10

      Dipetalonema perstans, D. streptocerca, Mansonella ozzardi   10

      Loa loa   11

      Onchocerca volvulus   12

      Dracunculus medinensis   13

Cestode worm

      Taenia solium   14

      Taenia saginata   15

      Hymenolepis nana, H. diminuta   16

      Dibothriocephalus latus   17

      Echinococcus granulosus   18

      Echinococcus multilocularis   19

            Pathology of Hydatid disease   19

Trematode worms

      Schistosoma spp : S. haematobium, S. mansoni, S. japonicum   20

            Pathology of Schistosomiasis   21

      Clonorchis sinensis   22

      Paragonimus westermani   23

      Fasciola hepatica   24

      Fasciolopsis buski   25

Recapitulation

      Morphology of adults and larvae   26-27

      Ova   28

      Routes of infection   29-30

PLATE 1

Initial classification of worms of medical importance.

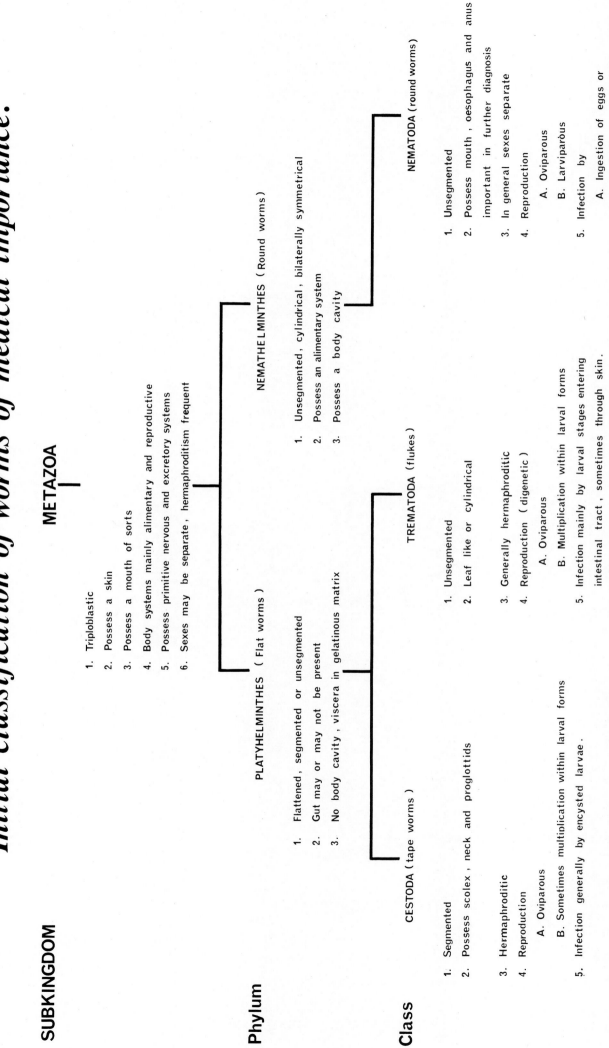

SUBKINGDOM METAZOA

1. Triploblastic
2. Possess a skin
3. Possess a mouth of sorts
4. Body systems mainly alimentary and reproductive
5. Possess primitive nervous and excretory systems
6. Sexes may be separate, hermaphroditism frequent

Phylum

PLATYHELMINTHES (Flat worms)

1. Flattened, segmented or unsegmented
2. Gut may or may not be present
3. No body cavity, viscera in gelatinous matrix

NEMATHELMINTHES (Round worms)

1. Unsegmented, cylindrical, bilaterally symmetrical
2. Possess an alimentary system
3. Possess a body cavity

Class

CESTODA (tape worms)

1. Segmented
2. Possess scolex , neck and proglottids
3. Hermaphroditic
4. Reproduction
   A. Oviparous
   B. Sometimes multiplication within larval forms
5. Infection generally by encysted larvae.

TREMATODA (flukes)

1. Unsegmented
2. Leaf like or cylindrical
3. Generally hermaphroditic
4. Reproduction (digenetic)
   A. Oviparous
   B. Multiplication within larval forms
5. Infection mainly by larval stages entering intestinal tract , sometimes through skin.

NEMATODA (round worms)

1. Unsegmented
2. Possess mouth , oesophagus and anus important in further diagnosis
3. In general sexes separate
4. Reproduction
   A. Oviparous
   B. Larviparous
5. Infection by
   A. Ingestion of eggs or
   B. Penetration of larvae through surfaces or
   C. Arthropod vector or
   D. Ingestion of encysted larvae.

PLATE 2

Ascaris lumbricoides (The round worm)

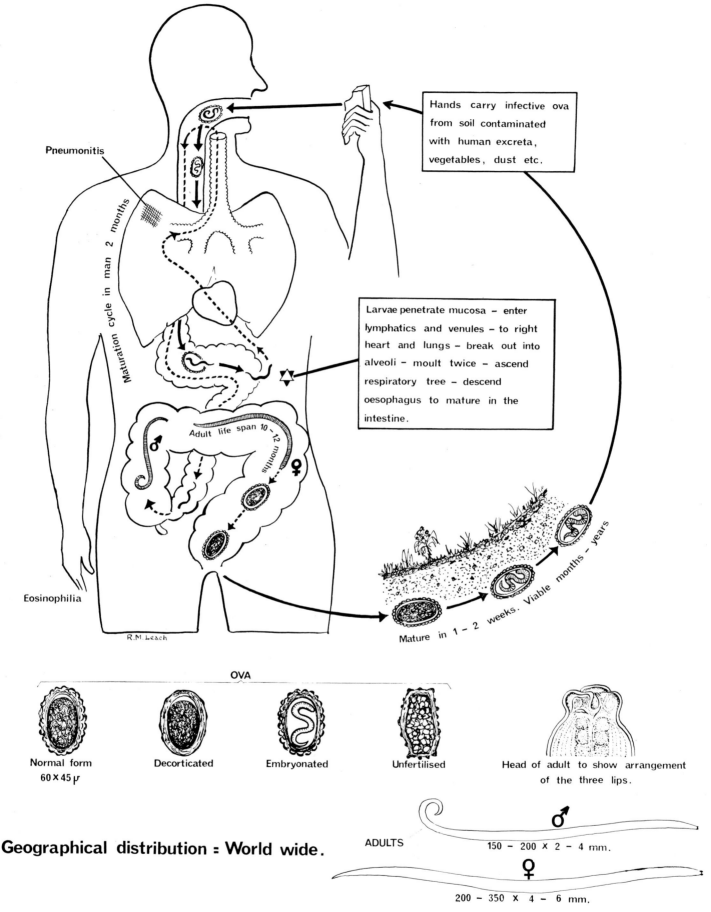

Pneumonitis

Maturation cycle in man 2 months

Hands carry infective ova from soil contaminated with human excreta, vegetables, dust etc.

Larvae penetrate mucosa – enter lymphatics and venules – to right heart and lungs – break out into alveoli – moult twice – ascend respiratory tree – descend oesophagus to mature in the intestine.

Adult life span 10 – 12 months

Eosinophilia

R.M.Leach

Mature in 1 – 2 weeks. Viable months – years

OVA

Normal form
60 × 45 μ

Decorticated

Embryonated

Unfertilised

Head of adult to show arrangement of the three lips.

ADULTS

♂ 150 – 200 × 2 – 4 mm.

♀ 200 – 350 × 4 – 6 mm.

Geographical distribution = World wide.

PATHOLOGY

LARVAE Allergy, eosinophilia and pneumonitis. Occasionally ectopic larvae in other organs with local inflammation and necrosis. (One form of larva migrans, see Plate 110.)

ADULTS Obstruction of intestine, bile ducts and trachea have been reported.

LABORATORY DIAGNOSIS

Recovery of ova from faeces. Rarely embryos may be found in sputum.

PLATE 3

Trichuris trichiura (The Whip worm)
Syn. Trichocephalus trichiura.

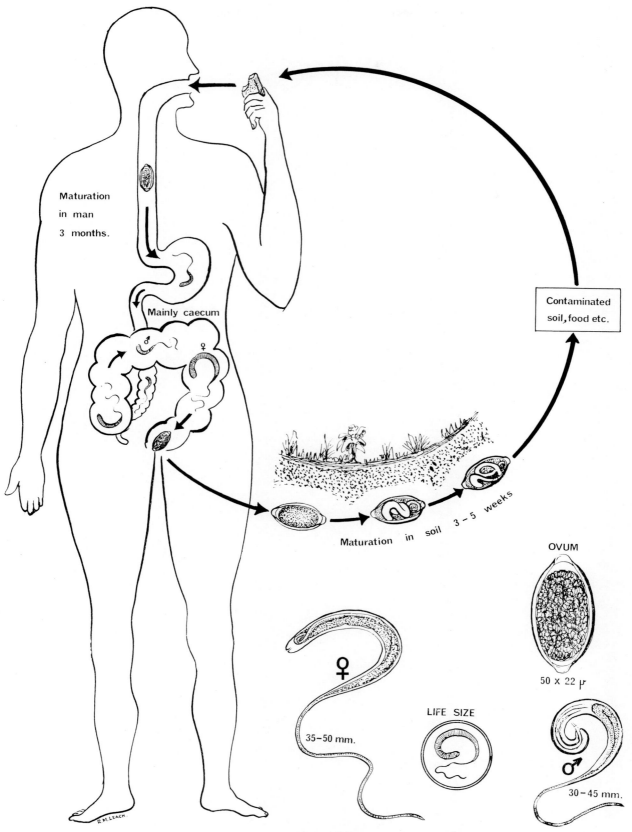

Maturation in man 3 months.

Mainly caecum

Contaminated soil, food etc.

Maturation in soil 3 - 5 weeks

OVUM

50 x 22 μ

♀

35 - 50 mm.

LIFE SIZE

♂

30 - 45 mm.

R.M.LEACH.

Geographical distribution = Cosmopolitan

PATHOLOGY

1. Generally none.
2. Very heavy infection – local inflammation – abdominal discomfort – diarrhoea – eosinophilia up to 25 %.

LABORATORY DIAGNOSIS

OVA in stools.

PLATE 4

Enterobius vermicularis. (Thread, pin or seat worm)
Syn. Oxyuris vermicularis.

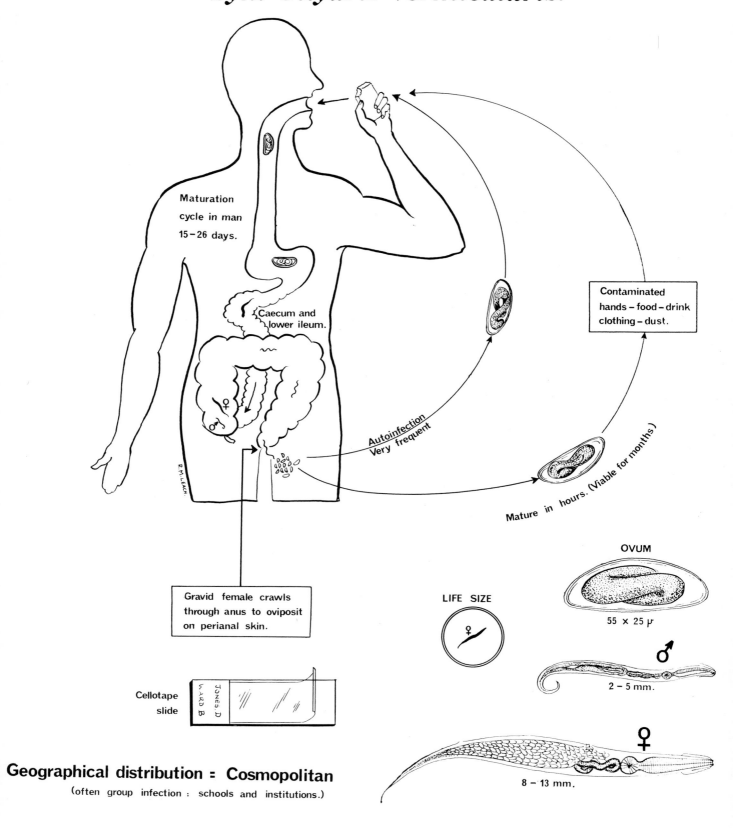

Geographical distribution = Cosmopolitan
(often group infection : schools and institutions.)

PATHOLOGY

1. Pruritus ani and vulvae.
2. Occasionally associated with obstructive appendicitis.
3. Eosinophilia up to 10%.

LABORATORY DIAGNOSIS

OVA in perianal scrapings.

in finger nail scrapings.

ADULTS in stool after purge or enema.

Strongyloides stercoralis

PLATE 5

Geographical distribution: Cosmopolitan
(Sporadic in temperate zones)

Rhabditiform larva
250 × 20 μ

Filariform larva
600 × 20 μ

Larvae mature in duodenum (or bronchus)

Fertilised ♀ enters mucosa, lays eggs which hatch to rhabditiform larvae, these then make their way to bowel lumen.

EOSINOPHILIA

Maturation stage in man 17 days

Enter circulation and via heart, lungs, respiratory tree and oesophagus reach intestine.

RHABDITIFORM LARVAE PASSED IN STOOL

RHABDITIFORM LARVAE METAMORPHOSE IN BOWEL TO FILARIFORM LARVAE

Survive weeks in soil

Fil

Rhab

Under unfavourable environmental conditions metamorphose to infective filariform larvae.

FREE LIVING

♂ & ♀

INDIRECT CYCLE

12-24 hrs

Moults

DIRECT CYCLE II

DIRECT CYCLE I

NEW HOST

SAME HOST SKIN

SAME HOST BOWEL WALL

AUTOINFECTION

HYPERINFECTION

PATHOLOGY

(1) INVASION OF BODY BY LARVAE

(a) Skin Local dermatitis

(b) Viscera Localised pneumonitis from migratory Larvae Occasionally ectopic larvae in brain and other viscera

(c) General Allergic reaction and eosinophilia

(a) Severe perianal dermatitis and larva migrans

(b) Severe pneumonitis and multiple ectopic larvae

(c) Severe general allergy occasionally fatal, eosinophilia

(2) INVASION OF BODY BY MATURE ADULTS

(a) May be some inflammation of intestinal mucosa producing diarrhoea

(b) Occasionally pneumonitis

(a) Severe mucosal inflammation and diarrhoea

(b) Severe pneumonitis more common

LABORATORY DIAGNOSIS·· Larvae in fresh faeces (occasionally in sputum)

PLATE 6

The Hookworms

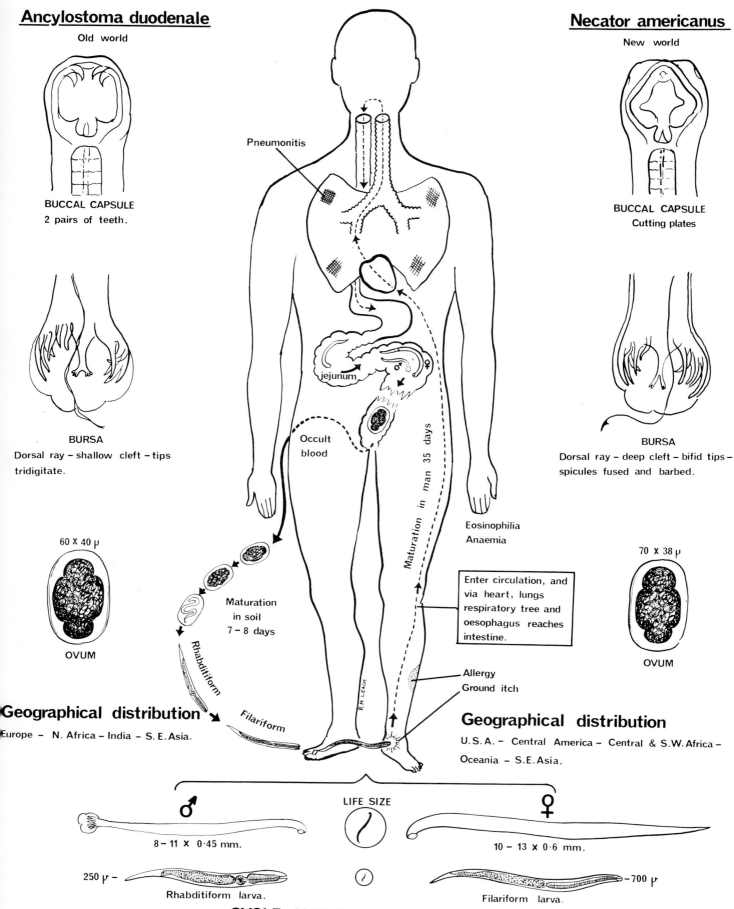

Ancylostoma duodenale
Old world

BUCCAL CAPSULE
2 pairs of teeth.

BURSA
Dorsal ray – shallow cleft – tips tridigitate.

60 X 40 μ

OVUM

Geographical distribution
Europe – N. Africa – India – S. E. Asia.

Necator americanus
New world

BUCCAL CAPSULE
Cutting plates

BURSA
Dorsal ray – deep cleft – bifid tips – spicules fused and barbed.

70 X 38 μ

OVUM

Geographical distribution
U.S.A. – Central America – Central & S.W. Africa – Oceania – S.E. Asia.

Pneumonitis

jejunum

Occult blood

Maturation in man 35 days

Eosinophilia
Anaemia

Enter circulation, and via heart, lungs respiratory tree and oesophagus reaches intestine.

Allergy
Ground itch

Maturation in soil 7 – 8 days

Rhabditiform

Filariform

♂ 8 – 11 X 0.45 mm.

LIFE SIZE

♀ 10 – 13 X 0.6 mm.

250 μ –   Rhabditiform larva.

– 700 μ   Filariform larva.

R.M.LEACH

CYCLE AND PATHOLOGY IN MAN

1. Infection   General allergic reactions – ground itch – cutaneous larva migrans in non-human ancylostomes.

2. Migration   Lung involvement – localised pneumonitis – eosinophilia – allergy.

3. Localisation In jejunum – ingestion of blood by parasites – occult bleeding from intestinal mucosa – anaemia (and sequelae).

LABORATORY DIAGNOSIS
Ova in stools.

PLATE 7

Trichinella spiralis

Cycle of development completed in single host (which is both definitive and intermediate.) Two hosts (carnivores) required to complete cycle.

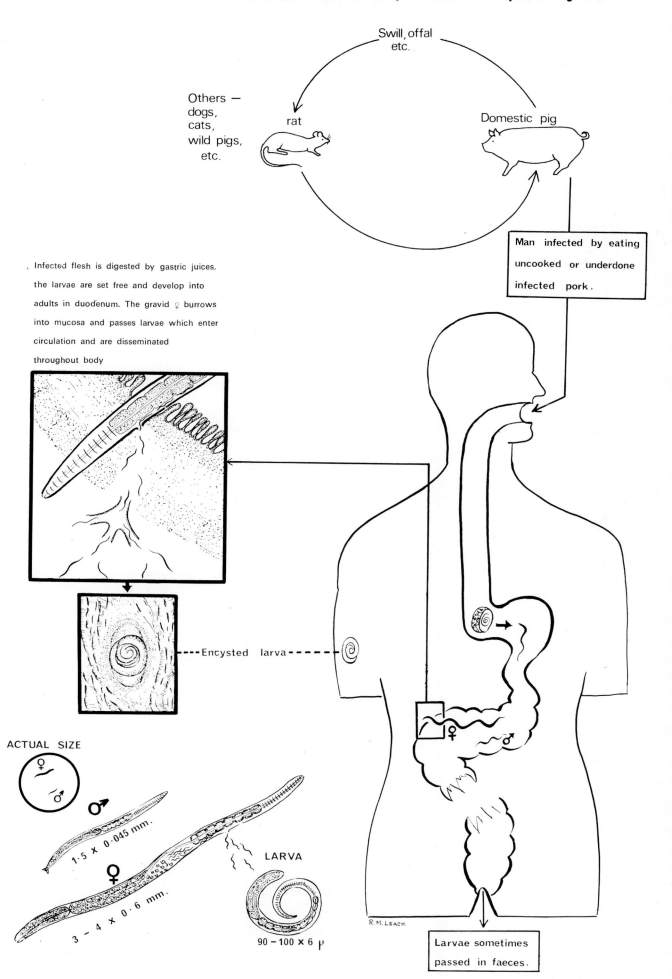

Swill, offal etc.

Others — dogs, cats, wild pigs, etc.

rat

Domestic pig

Man infected by eating uncooked or underdone infected pork.

Infected flesh is digested by gastric juices, the larvae are set free and develop into adults in duodenum. The gravid ♀ burrows into mucosa and passes larvae which enter circulation and are disseminated throughout body

- - - Encysted larva - - - - -

ACTUAL SIZE

♂ 1·5 x 0·045 mm.

♀ 3 - 4 x 0·6 mm.

LARVA

90 - 100 x 6 µ

R.M.LEACH.

Larvae sometimes passed in faeces.

Geographical distribution = Cosmopolitan (frequent in temperate climates).

CONTINUED ON PLATE 8

Trichinella spiralis

PLATE 8

CYCLE

PATHOLOGY

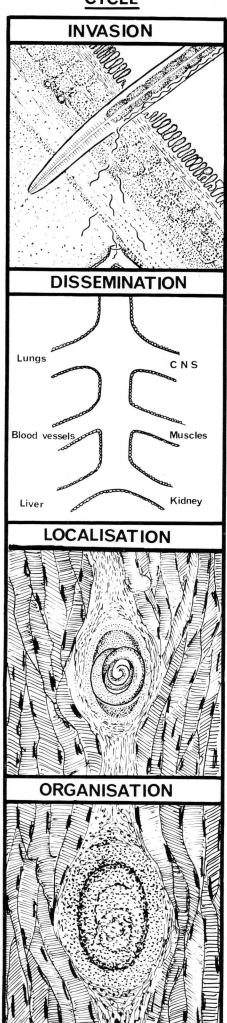

INVASION

DISSEMINATION

Lungs

CNS

Blood vessels

Muscles

Liver

Kidney

LOCALISATION

ORGANISATION

CYCLE

R.M.LEACH

INTESTINAL INFLAMMATION
ALLERGY.

GRANULOMATOUS REACTIONS
ANYWHERE BUT FURTHER
LARVAL DEVELOPMENT ONLY
IN STRIATED MUSCLE.

ESPECIALLY MUSCLES OF
RESPIRATION, TONGUE,
EYE.
DEGENERATION AND CELLULAR
INFILTRATION.

FIBROSIS (AND CALCIFICATION)

LABORATORY DIAGNOSIS

Diarrhoea stage.	Occasionally adults and / or larvae found in faeces
Encystment stage.	Muscle biopsy (Digestion or histology)
	Bachman intradermal test } Antigen − trichinal cyst Precipitin test on serum } extract.

PLATE 9

Wuchereria bancrofti

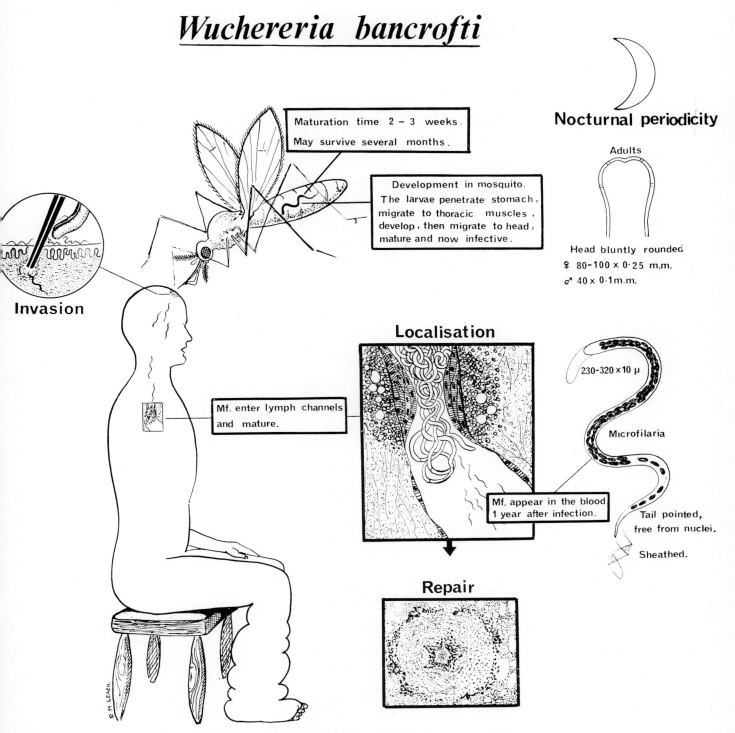

Nocturnal periodicity

Maturation time 2 – 3 weeks.
May survive several months.

Development in mosquito.
The larvae penetrate stomach,
migrate to thoracic muscles,
develop, then migrate to head,
mature and now infective.

Adults

Head bluntly rounded
♀ 80-100 x 0·25 m.m.
♂ 40 x 0·1 m.m.

Invasion

Mf. enter lymph channels
and mature.

Localisation

230-320 x 10 μ

Microfilaria

Mf. appear in the blood
1 year after infection.

Tail pointed,
free from nuclei.

Sheathed.

Repair

Geographical distribution = Asia, Africa, S. America, Australasia.

PATHOLOGY.

Adults in lymphatic channels cause —:

1. Proliferation of lining endothelium,

2. Surrounding infiltration of Eosinophils

Eosinophils		Obstruction	Lymph varices
Macrophages	Filarial granulation	Secondary infection	Lymphadenopathy
Lymphocytes	tissue leading to	Fibrosis	Elephantiasis
Giant cells		Calcification	Hydrocele, Chyluria etc.

LABORATORY DIAGNOSIS.

1. Microfilariæ in thick blood film (10 pm – 2 am) stained, unstained (centrifuge concentration). Chylous exudate or chylous urine.

2. Histological examination of biopsy material.

3. Intradermal test with dirofilarial antigen (only group – specific).

PLATE 10

Brugia malayi

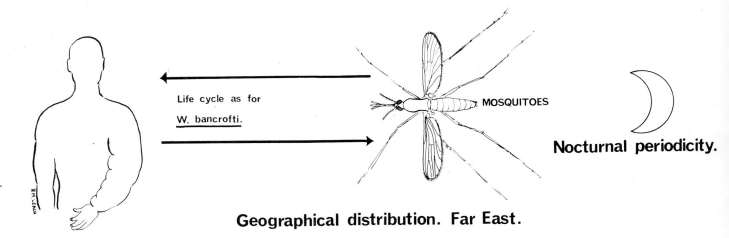

Life cycle as for W. bancrofti.

MOSQUITOES

Nocturnal periodicity.

Geographical distribution. Far East.

ADULTS	MICROFILARIA

Morphology

Resemble W. bancrofti

MICROFILARIA

170 – 260 × 5–6 µ

Sheathed

Two discrete nuclei in tip of tail.

PATHOLOGY

AS FOR W. BANCROFTI.

LABORATORY DIAGNOSIS

AS FOR W. BANCROFTI.

Other filarial worms.

Microfilariæ of other species may be found in the blood and tissues. These worms appear to be non-pathogenic and differentiation of microfilariæ from Wuchereria and Brugia necessary.

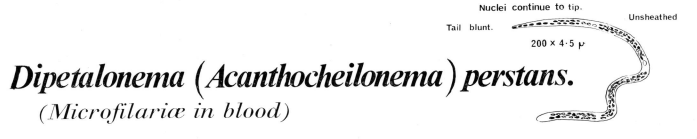

Nuclei continue to tip.

Tail blunt.

Unsheathed

200 × 4·5 µ

Dipetalonema (Acanthocheilonema) perstans.
(Microfilariæ in blood)

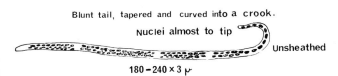

Blunt tail, tapered and curved into a crook.

Nuclei almost to tip

Unsheathed

180 – 240 × 3 µ

Dipetalonema streptocerca.
(Microfilariæ in skin)

Unsheathed

Tip of tail free of nuclei.

Mansonella ozzardi.
(Microfilariæ in blood)

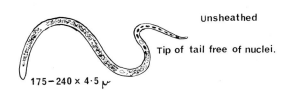

175 – 240 × 4·5 µ

PLATE 11

Loa loa (The eye worm)

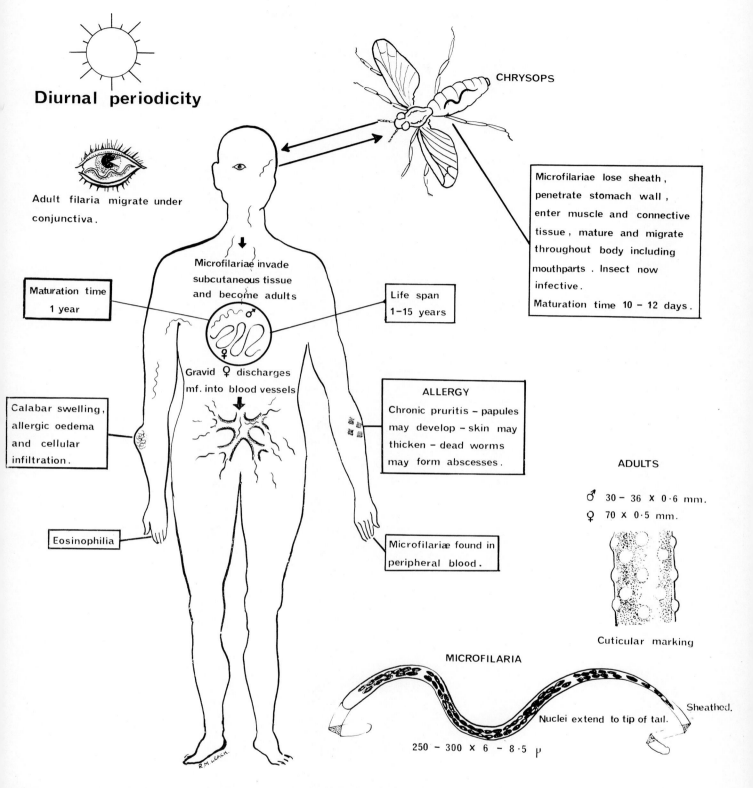

Diurnal periodicity

CHRYSOPS

Adult filaria migrate under conjunctiva.

Microfilariae invade subcutaneous tissue and become adults

Microfilariae lose sheath, penetrate stomach wall, enter muscle and connective tissue, mature and migrate throughout body including mouthparts. Insect now infective.
Maturation time 10 – 12 days.

Maturation time 1 year

Life span 1–15 years

Gravid ♀ discharges mf. into blood vessels

Calabar swelling, allergic oedema and cellular infiltration.

ALLERGY
Chronic pruritis – papules may develop – skin may thicken – dead worms may form abscesses.

ADULTS

♂ 30 – 36 x 0·6 mm.
♀ 70 x 0·5 mm.

Eosinophilia

Microfilariæ found in peripheral blood.

Cuticular marking

MICROFILARIA

Sheathed.

Nuclei extend to tip of tail.

250 – 300 x 6 – 8·5 µ

Geographical distribution = Equatorial, West and Central Africa.

PATHOLOGY.

Transient subcutaneous (calabar) swellings. Occasionally abscesses follow.
Eosinophilia (30 – 80 %).
Adult may appear under conjunctiva.

LABORATORY DIAGNOSIS.

Microfilariæ in blood.
Occasionally adult seen under conjunctiva or by biopsy of swelling.
Complement fixation or intradermal tests with dirofilarial antigen (group, not species, specific).

PLATE 12

Onchocerca volvulus
(The blinding worm)

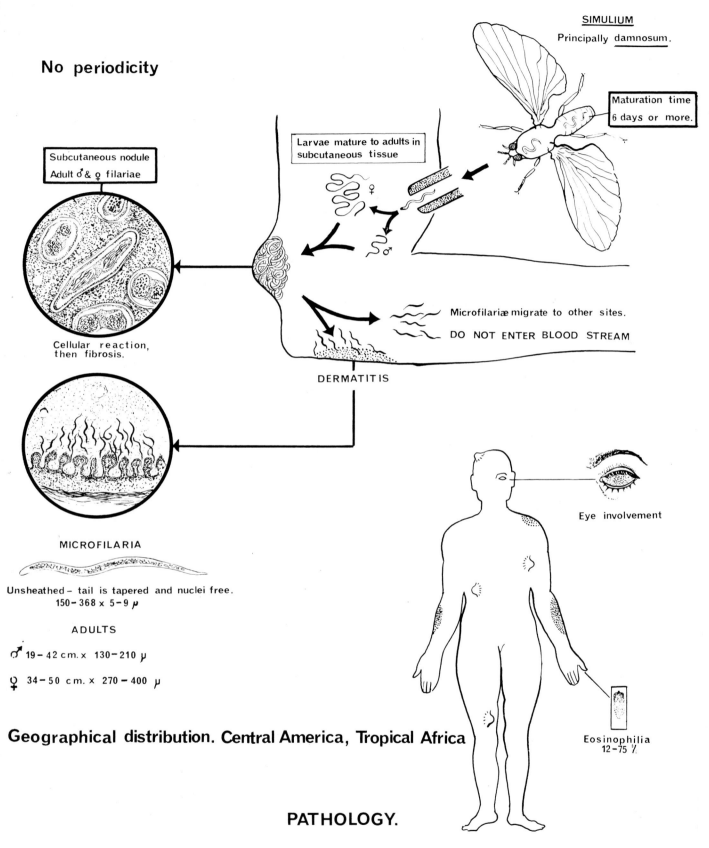

SIMULIUM
Principally damnosum.

No periodicity

Maturation time
6 days or more.

Larvae mature to adults in
subcutaneous tissue

Subcutaneous nodule
Adult ♂ & ♀ filariae

Cellular reaction,
then fibrosis.

Microfilariæ migrate to other sites.
DO NOT ENTER BLOOD STREAM

DERMATITIS

Eye involvement

MICROFILARIA

Unsheathed – tail is tapered and nuclei free.
150 – 368 x 5 – 9 μ

ADULTS

♂ 19 – 42 cm. x 130 – 210 μ

♀ 34 – 50 c.m. x 270 – 400 μ

Geographical distribution. Central America, Tropical Africa

Eosinophilia
12 – 75 %

PATHOLOGY.

Fibrous nodules develop round adults

Sometimes lymphatic obstruction. (Elephantiasis) In Africa

Dermatitis from microfilariae

Inflammatory lesions of eye invaded by microfilariae

Allergic reactions (Eosinophilia, Urticaria)

LABORATORY DIAGNOSIS

Detection of adults in excised nodules

Microfilariae in shavings of skin

(Serological tests of little value)

Dracunculus medinensis (The Guinea worm)

PLATE 13

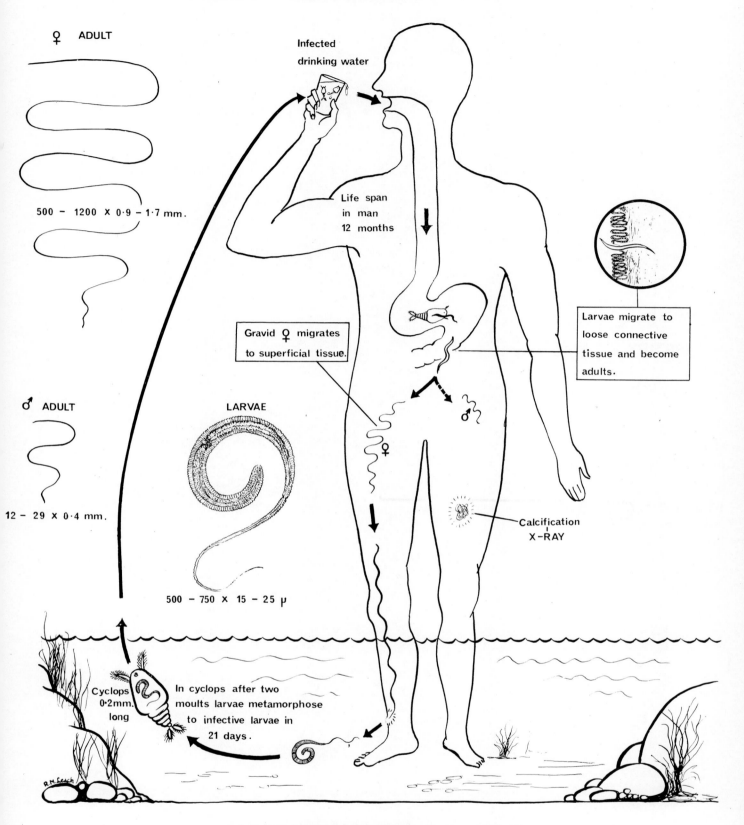

♀ ADULT

500 – 1200 X 0.9 – 1.7 mm.

Infected drinking water

Life span in man 12 months

Gravid ♀ migrates to superficial tissue.

Larvae migrate to loose connective tissue and become adults.

♂ ADULT

12 – 29 X 0.4 mm.

LARVAE

500 – 750 X 15 – 25 μ

Calcification X-RAY

Cyclops 0.2mm. long

In cyclops after two moults larvae metamorphose to infective larvae in 21 days.

R.M.Leach.

Geographical distribution = Africa, Asia.

PATHOLOGY

Migration of gravid female – allergy, eosinophilia.

Local lesion – papule – ulcer with discharge of embryos – fibrosis.

Secondary bacterial infection often.

LABORATORY DIAGNOSIS.

Larvae in fluid from ulcer.

PLATE 14

Taenia solium
(The pork tape worm)

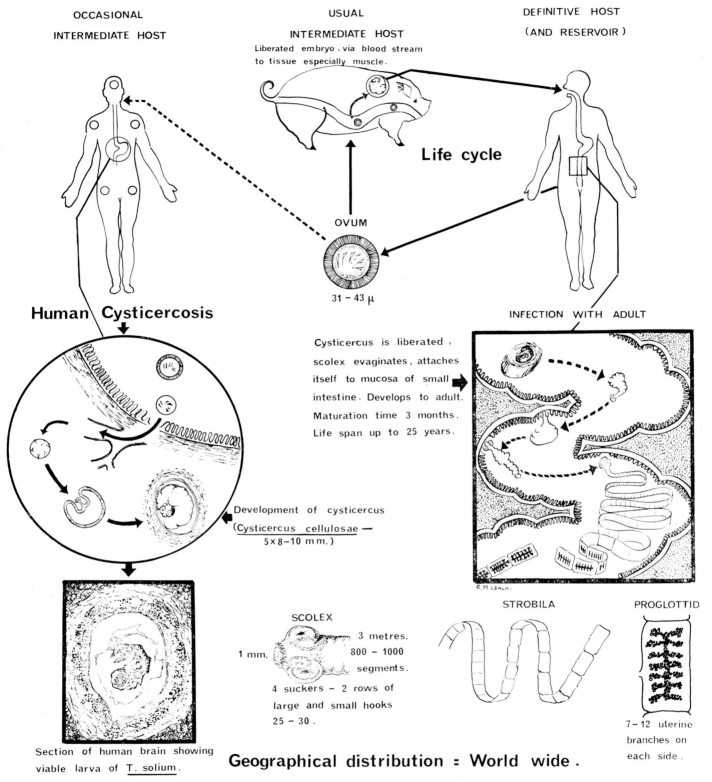

OCCASIONAL INTERMEDIATE HOST

USUAL INTERMEDIATE HOST

Liberated embryo, via blood stream to tissue especially muscle.

DEFINITIVE HOST (AND RESERVOIR)

Life cycle

OVUM

31 – 43 μ

Human Cysticercosis

Cysticercus is liberated, scolex evaginates, attaches itself to mucosa of small intestine. Develops to adult. Maturation time 3 months. Life span up to 25 years.

INFECTION WITH ADULT

Development of cysticercus (Cysticercus cellulosae — 5 x 8–10 m m.)

R. M. LEACH.

Section of human brain showing viable larva of T. solium.

SCOLEX

1 mm.

3 metres.
800 – 1000 segments.
4 suckers – 2 rows of large and small hooks 25 – 30.

STROBILA

PROGLOTTID

7 – 12 uterine branches on each side.

Geographical distribution = World wide.

PATHOLOGY.

INFECTION WITH LARVAE (CYSTICERCOSIS).

  Cysticerci may occur in any site, generally multiple, more frequent in brain and muscle

  Excite reaction around especially when they die
    Inflammation
    Fibrosis
    Later sometimes calcification
  Leading mainly to
    Focal CNS syndromes (eg epilepsy)
    Blood eosinophilia (10 ⁒) .

INFECTION WITH ADULTS.
  Often none
  Mild irritation of intestinal mucosa
  Eosinophilia up to 25⁒ .

LABORATORY DIAGNOSIS

  Histological examination, biopsy material.
  Gravid segments ⎫
  Ova   ⎬ in faeces
  Scolex   ⎭

PLATE 15

Taenia saginata
(The beef tape worm)

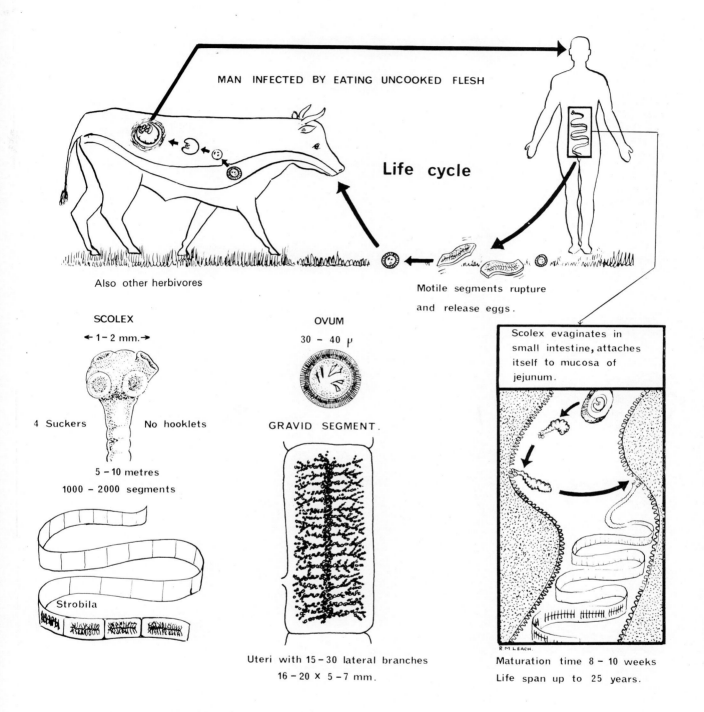

MAN INFECTED BY EATING UNCOOKED FLESH

Life cycle

Also other herbivores

Motile segments rupture
and release eggs.

SCOLEX

← 1 – 2 mm. →

4 Suckers   No hooklets

5 – 10 metres
1000 – 2000 segments

Strobila

OVUM

30 – 40 μ

GRAVID SEGMENT.

Uteri with 15 – 30 lateral branches
16 – 20 × 5 – 7 mm.

Scolex evaginates in
small intestine, attaches
itself to mucosa of
jejunum.

Maturation time 8 – 10 weeks
Life span up to 25 years.

Geographical distribution = world wide.

PATHOLOGY.

Usually none (Cysticercus bovis practically unknown in man.)

Occasionally vague alimentary upset.

Eosinophilia up to 10 / .

LABORATORY DIAGNOSIS.

Gravid segments
Ova   } in faeces.
Scolex

Ova on perianal skin (cellotape slide)

DWARF TAPEWORMS

Hymenolepis nana

PLATE 16

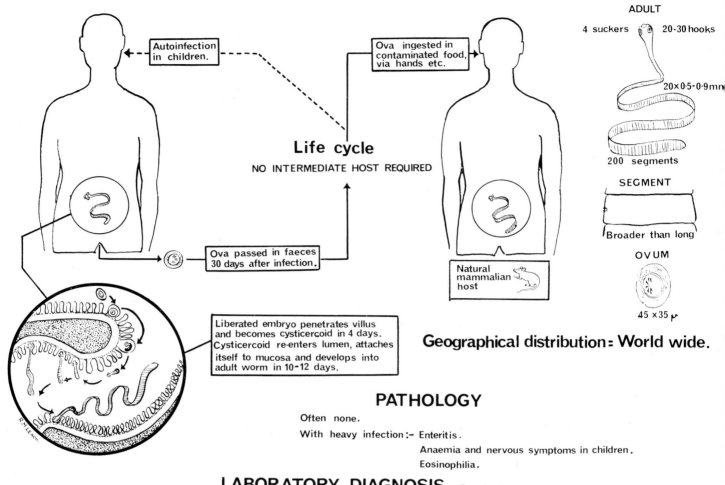

ADULT

4 suckers 20-30 hooks

20 × 0.5 - 0.9 mm

200 segments

SEGMENT

Broader than long

OVUM

45 × 35 µ

Autoinfection in children.

Ova ingested in contaminated food, via hands etc.

Life cycle
NO INTERMEDIATE HOST REQUIRED

Ova passed in faeces 30 days after infection.

Natural mammalian host

Liberated embryo penetrates villus and becomes cysticercoid in 4 days. Cysticercoid re-enters lumen, attaches itself to mucosa and develops into adult worm in 10-12 days.

Geographical distribution = World wide.

PATHOLOGY

Often none.

With heavy infection :- Enteritis.
Anaemia and nervous symptoms in children.
Eosinophilia.

LABORATORY DIAGNOSIS. Ova in faeces.

Hymenolepis diminuta.

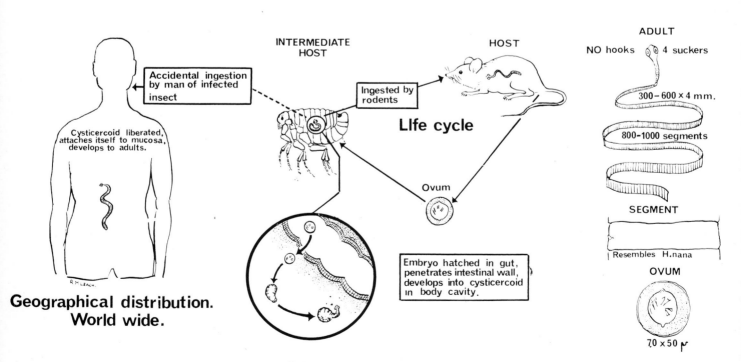

ADULT

NO hooks 4 suckers

300 - 600 × 4 mm.

800-1000 segments

SEGMENT

Resembles H. nana

OVUM

70 × 50 µ

INTERMEDIATE HOST

HOST

Accidental ingestion by man of infected insect

Ingested by rodents

Life cycle

Cysticercoid liberated, attaches itself to mucosa, develops to adults.

Ovum

Embryo hatched in gut, penetrates intestinal wall, develops into cysticercoid in body cavity.

Geographical distribution. World wide.

PATHOLOGY

Incidence in man low.
Generally no effect on host.

LABORATORY DIAGNOSIS

Ova in faeces.

PLATE 17

Dibothriocephalus latus

Syn. Diphyllobothrium latum (broad or fish tape worm).

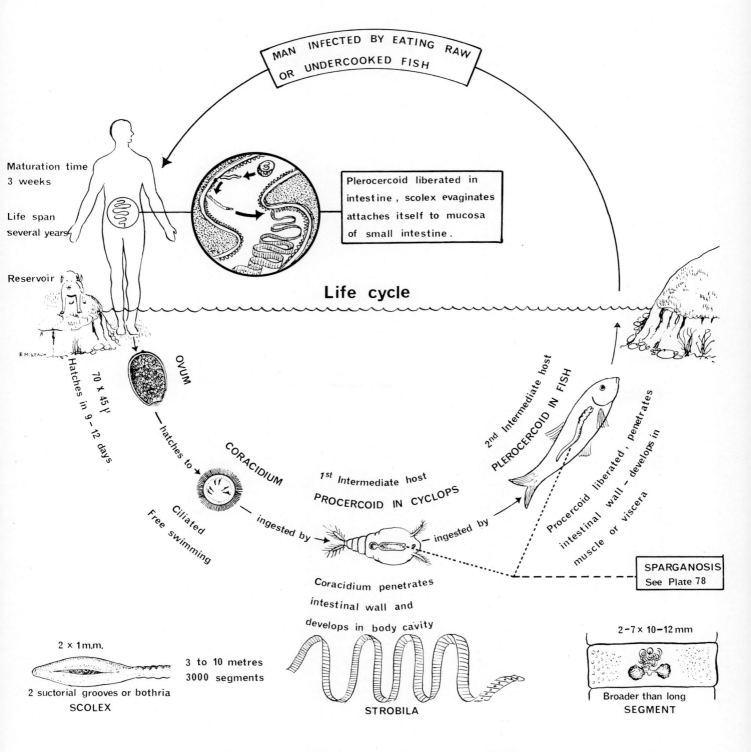

MAN INFECTED BY EATING RAW OR UNDERCOOKED FISH

Maturation time 3 weeks

Life span several years

Reservoir

R.M.LEACH

Plerocercoid liberated in intestine, scolex evaginates attaches itself to mucosa of small intestine.

Life cycle

70 x 45 µ
Hatches in 9 – 12 days

OVUM

hatches to

CORACIDIUM

Ciliated
Free swimming

ingested by

1st Intermediate host
PROCERCOID IN CYCLOPS

ingested by

2nd Intermediate host
PLEROCERCOID IN FISH

Procercoid liberated, penetrates intestinal wall – develops in muscle or viscera

Coracidium penetrates intestinal wall and develops in body cavity

SPARGANOSIS
See Plate 78

2 x 1 m.m.

3 to 10 metres
3000 segments

2 suctorial grooves or bothria
SCOLEX

STROBILA

2–7 x 10–12 mm

Broader than long
SEGMENT

Geographical distribution : Europe, Asia, America.

PATHOLOGY

Generally none.

Occasionally macrocytic anaemia (absorption of B 12 by worm).

LABORATORY DIAGNOSIS

Eggs in faeces

Echinococcus granulosus

PLATE 18

(Causing Hydatid disease)

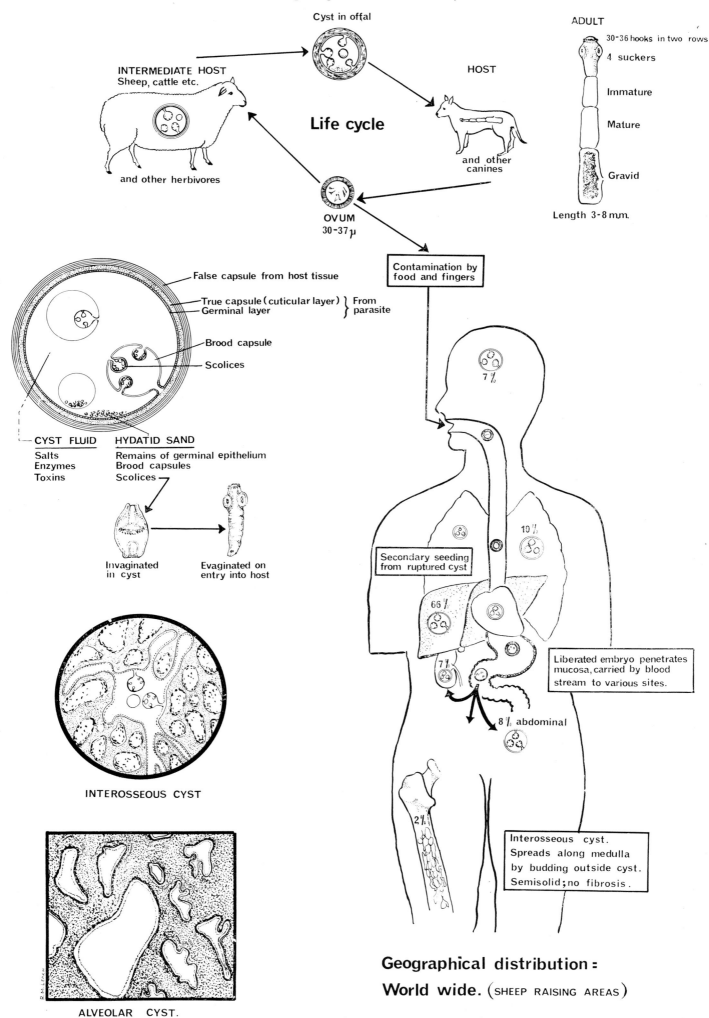

Cyst in offal

ADULT

INTERMEDIATE HOST
Sheep, cattle etc.

HOST

30-36 hooks in two rows
4 suckers

Immature

Mature

Gravid

Length 3-8 m.m.

Life cycle

and other herbivores

and other canines

OVUM
30-37 μ

Contamination by food and fingers

False capsule from host tissue

True capsule (cuticular layer) } From
Germinal layer } parasite

Brood capsule

Scolices

7 %

CYST FLUID
Salts
Enzymes
Toxins

HYDATID SAND
Remains of germinal epithelium
Brood capsules
Scolices

Invaginated in cyst

Evaginated on entry into host

Secondary seeding from ruptured cyst

10 %

66 %

7 %

Liberated embryo penetrates mucosa, carried by blood stream to various sites.

8 % abdominal

INTEROSSEOUS CYST

2 %

Interosseous cyst.
Spreads along medulla by budding outside cyst.
Semisolid; no fibrosis.

Geographical distribution =
World wide. (SHEEP RAISING AREAS)

ALVEOLAR CYST.

Probably related species E. multilocularis.

CONTINUED ON PLATE 19.

Echinococcus multilocularis

PLATE 19

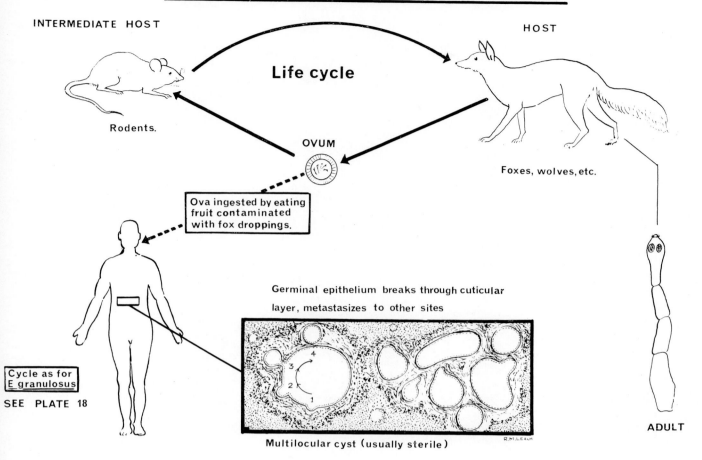

INTERMEDIATE HOST

HOST

Life cycle

Rodents.

OVUM

Foxes, wolves, etc.

Ova ingested by eating fruit contaminated with fox droppings.

Germinal epithelium breaks through cuticular layer, metastasizes to other sites

Cycle as for E granulosus

SEE PLATE 18

Multilocular cyst (usually sterile)

ADULT

Geographical distribution: chiefly Russia, Siberia, Bavaria, The Tyrol and North America (especially Canada and Alaska)

PATHOLOGY OF HYDATID DISEASE.

1. UNILOCULAR CYSTS
   a) Surrounding inflammatory reaction and fibrosis
      After years may die, shrink, calcify.
   b) General allergy – eosinophilia, asthma etc.
   c) Pressure effects – local tissue damage
      obstruction of natural channels.
   d) Leakage or rupture – allergy accentuated
      anaphylactic shock sometimes
      secondary implantation (eg. peritoneal).
   e) Secondary infection with abscess formation.

2. OSSEUS CYSTS
   a) No fibrosis (some cellular infiltration)
   b) Bone destruction sometimes leading to
   c) Spontaneous fracture.

3. ALVEOLAR CYSTS
   a) Local pressure effects
   b) Allergy
   c) Germinal epithelium acts like a neoplasm with
      local infiltration or
      distant metastases.

LABORATORY DIAGNOSIS OF HYDATID DISEASE.

1. Casoni's intradermal test.
2. Serological tests eg. complement fixation on serum or C S F.
3. Histological examination of removed specimen
   (note : aspiration or partial biopsy may lead to anaphylaxis or secondary infection)

Schistosoma species
(The blood flukes)

PLATE 20

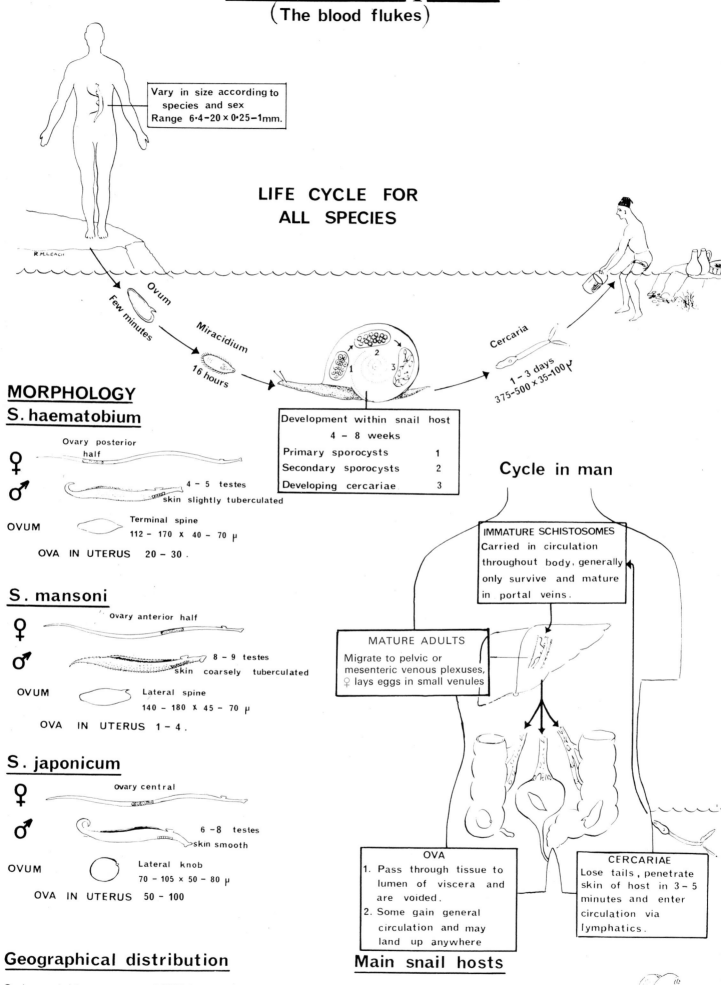

Vary in size according to species and sex
Range 6·4–20 × 0·25–1mm.

LIFE CYCLE FOR ALL SPECIES

R.M.LEACH

Ovum

Few minutes

Miracidium

16 hours

Cercaria

1 – 3 days
375–500 × 35–100 µ

Development within snail host
4 – 8 weeks

Primary sporocysts	1
Secondary sporocysts	2
Developing cercariae	3

MORPHOLOGY

S. haematobium

♀ Ovary posterior half

♂ 4 – 5 testes
skin slightly tuberculated

OVUM Terminal spine
112 – 170 × 40 – 70 µ

OVA IN UTERUS 20 – 30.

S. mansoni

♀ Ovary anterior half

♂ 8 – 9 testes
skin coarsely tuberculated

OVUM Lateral spine
140 – 180 × 45 – 70 µ

OVA IN UTERUS 1 – 4.

S. japonicum

♀ Ovary central

♂ 6 – 8 testes
skin smooth

OVUM Lateral knob
70 – 105 × 50 – 80 µ

OVA IN UTERUS 50 – 100

Cycle in man

IMMATURE SCHISTOSOMES
Carried in circulation throughout body, generally only survive and mature in portal veins.

MATURE ADULTS
Migrate to pelvic or mesenteric venous plexuses, ♀ lays eggs in small venules

OVA
1. Pass through tissue to lumen of viscera and are voided.
2. Some gain general circulation and may land up anywhere

CERCARIAE
Lose tails, penetrate skin of host in 3 – 5 minutes and enter circulation via lymphatics.

Geographical distribution

S. haematobium — AFRICA to IRAN.

S. mansoni — AFRICA , S. AMERICA

S. japonicum — FAR EAST

Main snail hosts

S. haematobium — Spp. of Bulinus

S. mansoni — Spp. of Biomphalaria , Australorbis

S. japonicum — Spp. of Oncomelania (operculate)

PLATE 21

Pathology of Schistosomiasis

General

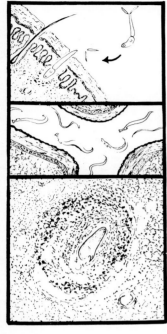

1. **PENETRATION OF SKIN BY CERCARIAE**.

   a) Pathogenic spp. Only slight local reaction (petechiae)

   b) Non – human spp. Cause **CERCARIAL DERMATITIS** (swimmer's itch)
   Papules – macules – vesicles – intense itching.

2. **MIGRATION OF IMMATURE WORMS**.

   General toxic and allergic symptoms (eosinophilia up to 50 %)

3. **DAMAGE BY EGGS IN TISSUE** (result depends on parasite load)

   Inflammatory reaction with epithelial ⎫
                              giant   ⎬ cells
                              plasma
                              eosinophil ⎭
                              fibroblasts

   Subsequent FIBROSIS and calcification.

4. **SEQUELAE OF SUCH DAMAGE — LOCAL — ECTOPIC**

Particular

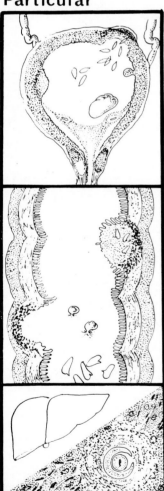

Urinary SCHISTOSOMIASIS (mainly due to S . haematobium)

1. Initial toxic and allergic symptoms not marked.

2. a) BLADDER and URETERS typically involved with

       Hyperaemia – papules – papillomata – ulceration

       Hypertrophy of bladder, later contraction

       Cystitis and calculus formation

       Development of fistulae

       Ova in urine

   b) GENITALIA and RENAL PELVIS sometimes affected , INTESTINE occasionally.

3. ECTOPIC lesions less severe than in other spp.

Intestinal SCHISTOSOMIASIS (S . mansoni)

1. Initial toxic and allergic symptoms marked.

2. a) LARGE INTESTINE and RECTUM typically involved with

       Papules – abscesses – ulcers – papillomata – fistulae – ova in faeces.

   b) BLADDER sometimes involved , pathology as for urinary type.

3. ECTOPIC lesions a) LIVER frequently involved (eggs via portal vein) with

       Inflammatory reaction ⎫
                           ⎬ leading to cirrhosis with ⎧ Portal hypertension
       Fibrosis   ⎭   ⎨ Splenomegaly
                                                              ⎩ Ascites

       b) ELSEWHERE (brain etc)

Oriental SCHISTOSOMIASIS (S . japonicum)

1. Initial toxic and allergic symptoms marked.

2. INTESTINAL lesions like mansoni infection , SMALL INTESTINE often involved.

3. ECTOPIC lesions a) LIVER frequently affected as in mansoni.

       b) BRAIN etc more frequent.

R.M.LEACH.

LABORATORY DIAGNOSIS

1. Ova in urine or faeces.

2. Ova in scrapings and biopsy material.

3. Intradermal test (antigen from infected snail liver).

4. Serological tests . Complement fixation.

PLATE 22

Clonorchis sinensis

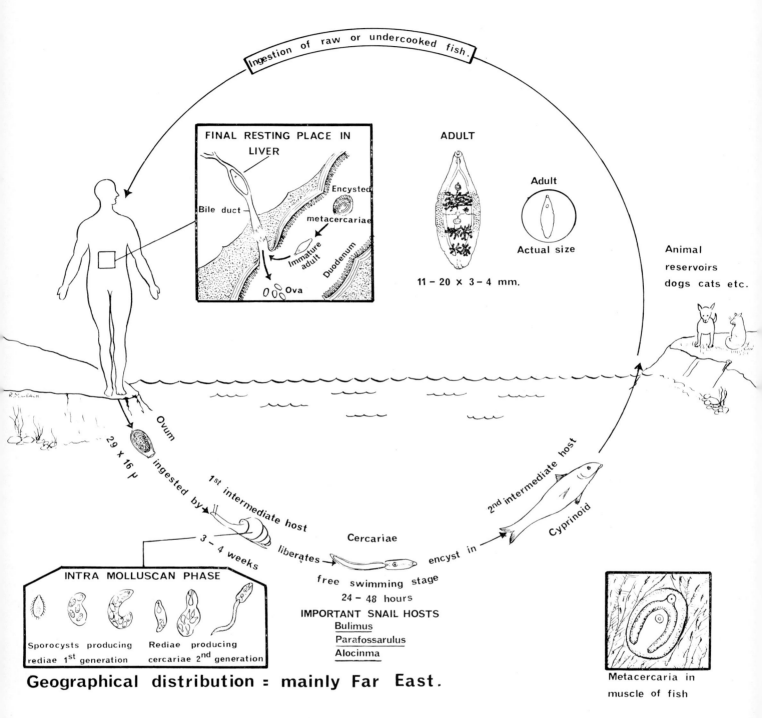

Geographical distribution = mainly Far East.

PATHOLOGY.

Adults inhabit distal bile ducts with –

    1. Epithelial proliferation.

    2. Surrounding inflammatory reaction.

    3. Sometimes secondary infection.

    4. Eosinophilia.

Leading to –

    1. .Thick , dilated fibrous ducts with adenomata of epithelium.

    2. Cirrhosis and destruction of liver parenchyma.

    3. Portal hypertension with splenomegaly.

Occasionally pancreatic ducts invaded with similar changes in pancreas.

LABORATORY DIAGNOSIS

    OVA   In faeces

             In bile (by duodenal tube)

Paragonimus westermani

(The lung fluke)

PLATE 23

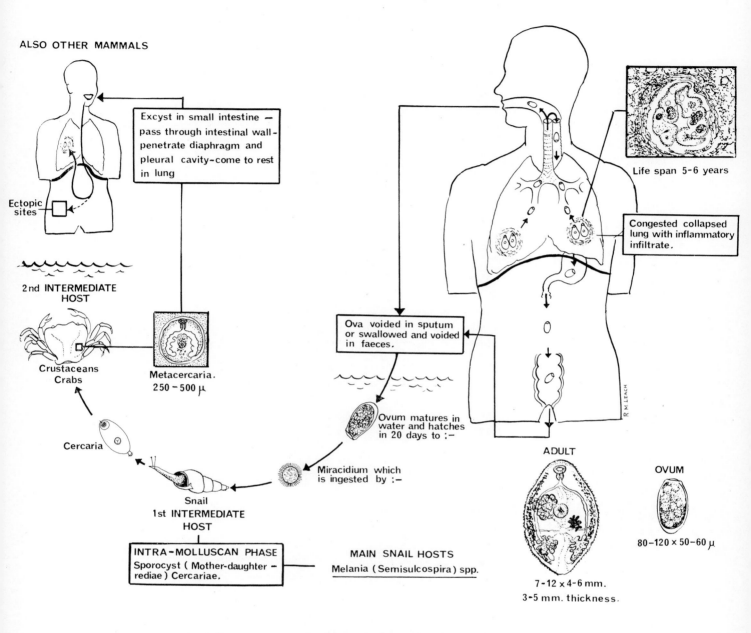

ALSO OTHER MAMMALS

Excyst in small intestine — pass through intestinal wall — penetrate diaphragm and pleural cavity — come to rest in lung

Ectopic sites

2nd INTERMEDIATE HOST

Crustaceans Crabs

Metacercaria. 250 – 500 μ

Cercaria

Snail
1st INTERMEDIATE HOST

INTRA-MOLLUSCAN PHASE
Sporocyst (Mother-daughter - rediae) Cercariae.

MAIN SNAIL HOSTS
Melania (Semisulcospira) spp.

Life span 5-6 years

Congested collapsed lung with inflammatory infiltrate.

Ova voided in sputum or swallowed and voided in faeces.

Ovum matures in water and hatches in 20 days to :-

Miracidium which is ingested by :-

ADULT

7-12 x 4-6 mm.
3-5 mm. thickness.

OVUM

80-120 × 50-60 μ

R M LEACH

Geographical distribution : Far East, S. America, Occasionally Africa.

PATHOLOGY

INVASION — Little effect on host

LOCALISATION IN LUNGS —
(1) Tissue reaction leading to formation of fibrous tissue capsule (slate blue in colour) containing –
      Worms (generally in pairs)
      Ova
      Inflammatory infiltration
      Connected with respiratory passages

(2) Secondary complications of lung cysts
      Bronchiectasis
      Abscess formation
      Tuberculosis frequent

LOCALISATION IN ECTOPIC SITES — Similar cysts may be found anywhere in body

GENERAL MANIFESTATIONS — Eosinophilia

LABORATORY DIAGNOSIS

OVA in sputum or faeces

Serological tests C F (extract of adult flukes as antigen)

Fasciola hepatica

PLATE 24

(The sheep liver fluke)

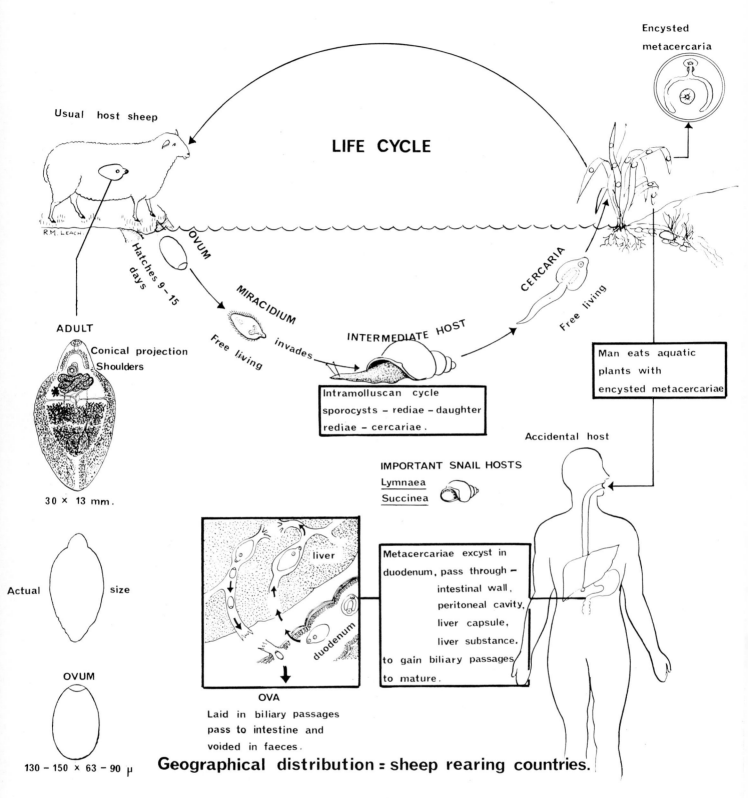

LIFE CYCLE

Encysted metacercaria

Usual host sheep

Hatches 9 – 15 days

OVUM

MIRACIDIUM Free living invades

INTERMEDIATE HOST

CERCARIA Free living

ADULT

Conical projection
Shoulders

30 × 13 mm.

Intramolluscan cycle
sporocysts – rediae – daughter
rediae – cercariae.

Man eats aquatic plants with encysted metacercariae

Accidental host

IMPORTANT SNAIL HOSTS
Lymnaea
Succinea

Actual size

liver

duodenum

Metacercariae excyst in
duodenum, pass through –
intestinal wall,
peritoneal cavity,
liver capsule,
liver substance.
to gain biliary passages
to mature.

OVUM

OVA
Laid in biliary passages
pass to intestine and
voided in faeces.

130 – 150 × 63 – 90 µ

Geographical distribution = sheep rearing countries.

PATHOLOGY.

(1) Transit of immature worms through liver. Mechanical and toxic irritation with – Toxaemia
                                                         Necrosis
                                                       Secondary fibrosis

(2) Development in bile ducts. – Cystic enlargement of ducts
                          Endothelial hyperplasia and adenomata
                          Secondary inflammatory infiltration — Fibrosis.

(3) Secondary bacterial infection. – Abscesses.

(4) Allergy. – (Eosinophilia.)

(5) Ectopic worms. – Lungs, brain, eyes, etc. with similar reactions.

(6) Pharyngeal infection. – (Halzoun) by adults, if infected raw sheep or goat livers eaten. Local irritation results.

LABORATORY DIAGNOSIS.

Ova in faeces. C F T (Cross reaction with F. buski.)

PLATE 25

Fasciolopsis buski

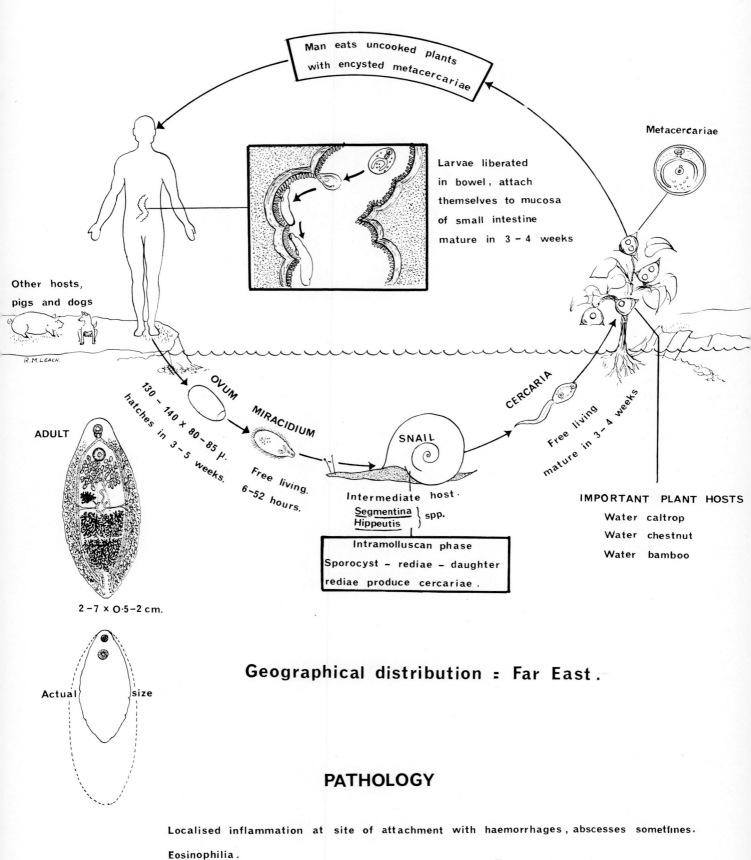

Man eats uncooked plants with encysted metacercariae

Metacercariae

Larvae liberated in bowel, attach themselves to mucosa of small intestine mature in 3 – 4 weeks

Other hosts, pigs and dogs

R.M.LEACH.

OVUM

130 – 140 x 80 – 85 μ.
hatches in 3 – 5 weeks.

MIRACIDIUM

Free living. 6–52 hours.

CERCARIA

Free living mature in 3 – 4 weeks

SNAIL

Intermediate host.
<u>Segmentina</u>
<u>Hippeutis</u> } spp.

Intramolluscan phase
Sporocyst – rediae – daughter rediae produce cercariae.

ADULT

2 – 7 x O·5–2 cm.

Actual   size

IMPORTANT PLANT HOSTS
Water caltrop
Water chestnut
Water bamboo

Geographical distribution = Far East.

PATHOLOGY

Localised inflammation at site of attachment with haemorrhages, abscesses sometimes.
Eosinophilia.

LABORATORY DIAGNOSIS

Ova, sometimes adults, in faeces.
C F T (Cross reaction with <u>F.hepatica.</u>)

Recapitulation
Morphology of adults and larvae.

PLATE 26

HEADS

A. lumbricoides

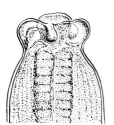

Three lips

E. vermicularis

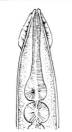

Bulbous oesophagus

NEMATODES

A. duodenale

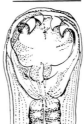

Buccal capsule with 2 pairs of teeth

N. americanus

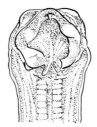

Buccal capsule with cutting plates

W. bancrofti

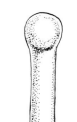

Bluntly rounded

TAILS

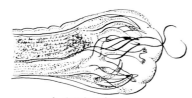

A. duodenale
Bursa with dorsal ray–shallow cleft –tips tridigitate

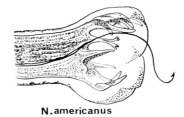

N. americanus
Bursa with dorsal ray– deep cleft – tips bifid. Spicule fused and barbed

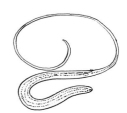

T. trichiura
Head attenuated from tail

LARVAE

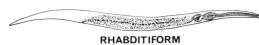

RHABDITIFORM
Bulbous oesophagus

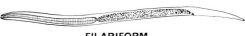

FILARIFORM
Straight oesophagus

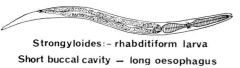

Strongyloides:– rhabditiform larva
Short buccal cavity — long oesophagus

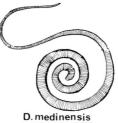

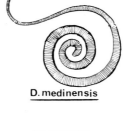

D. medinensis

Ancylostome:–rhabditiform larva
Long buccal cavity–short oesophagus

MICROFILARIA SHEATHED

W. bancrofti

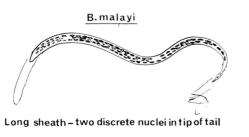

Nuclei do not reach tip of tail

Loa loa

Nuclei reach tip of tail

B. malayi

Long sheath – two discrete nuclei in tip of tail

IN TISSUE

T. spiralis in muscle

O. volvulus in subcutaneous tissue

MICROFILARIA UNSHEATHED

D. perstans

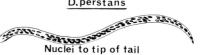

Nuclei to tip of tail

M. ozzardi

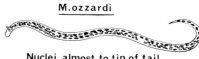

Nuclei almost to tip of tail

D. streptocerca

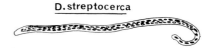

Tail blunt – curved like "shepherds crook"

O. volvulus

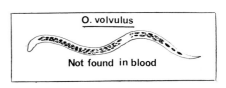

Not found in blood

R.M.LEACH

Heads

CESTODES

T.solium	T.saginata	H.nana	H.diminuta	D.latum	E.granulosus

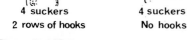

4 suckers	4 suckers	4 suckers	4 suckers	Suctorial grooves	(Larval form)
2 rows of hooks	No hooks	20-30 hooks	No hooks		4 suckers
					30-36 hooks

Proglottides

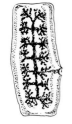
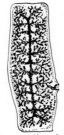
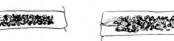
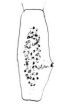

Uterus coiled

← Broader than long →

Longer than broad	Longer than broad				Adult in dogs
7-12 uterine branches each side	15-30 uterine branches each side				

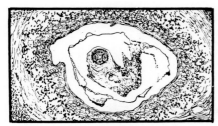

Cysticercosis.   Larval form of T.solium

In tissues

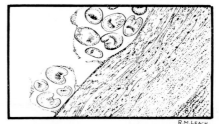

Hydatid cyst.   Larval forms of E.granulosus

R.M.LEACH.

TREMATODES

S.haematobium	S.mansoni	S.japonicum
Skin finely tuberculated 4-5 testes	Skin coarsely tuberculated 8-9 testes	Skin smooth 6-8 testes
♂	♂	♂
♀	♀	♀
Ovary posterior	Ovary anterior	Ovary central

Cercaria

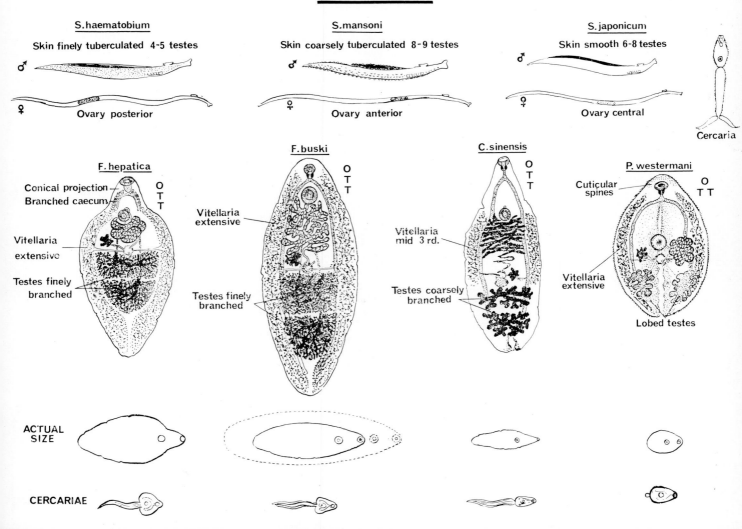

F. hepatica — Conical projection, Branched caecum, Vitellaria extensive, Testes finely branched — O T T

F.buski — Vitellaria extensive, Testes finely branched — O T T

C.sinensis — Vitellaria mid 3 rd., Testes coarsely branched — O T T

P. westermani — Cuticular spines, Vitellaria extensive, Lobed testes — O T T

ACTUAL SIZE

CERCARIAE

PLATE 28

Recapitulation *Ova*

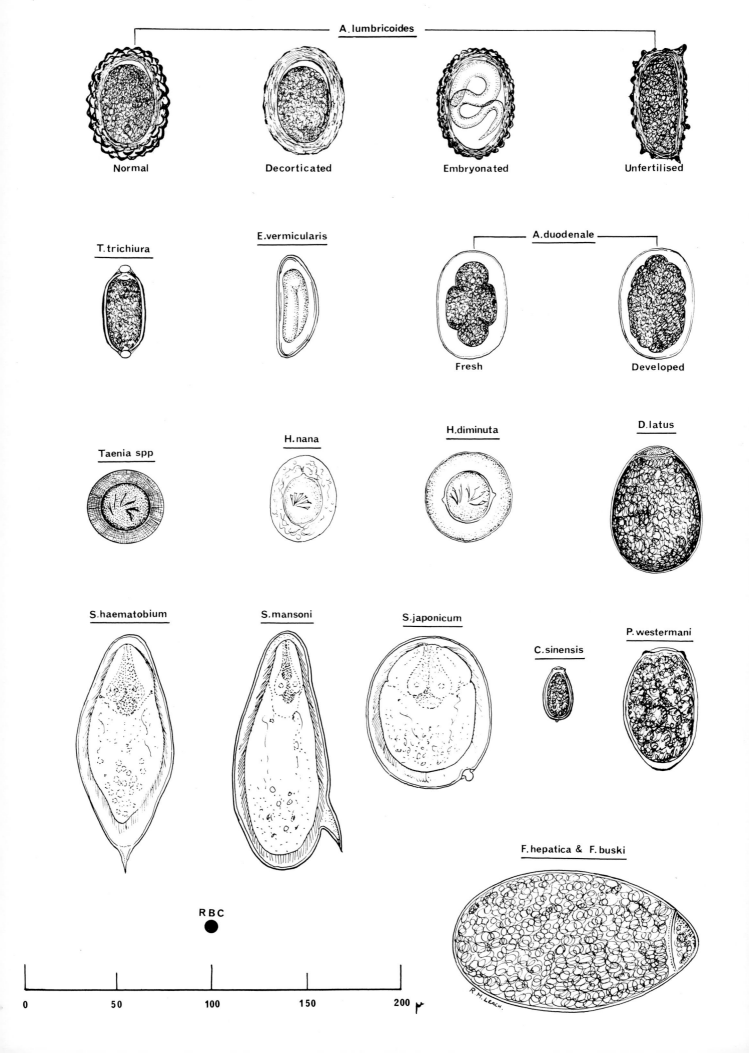

Recapitulation

PLATE 29

ROUTES OF INFECTION : THE KEY TO PREVENTION

HUMAN INFECTION BY	ROUTE OUTSIDE BODY	CLASS	SPECIES	PLATE
INGESTING OVA	INFECTIVE ova voided in faeces To new or same host on FINGERS, in DUST etc.	Nematoda	Enterobius vermicularis	4
		Cestoda	Hymenolepis nana	16
			Taenia solium (in human cysticercosis)	14
			Echinococcus granulosus (in hydatid disease)	18
	IMMATURE ova voided in faeces MATURE in SOIL To new host on VEGETABLES etc.	Nematoda	Trichuris trichiura	3
			Ascaris lumbricoides	2
PENETRATION OF SKIN BY LARVAE (a) from SOIL	Ova voided in faeces HATCH in SOIL Rhabditiform then filariform larvae (infective)	Nematoda	Ancylostoma duodenale	6
			Necator americanus	6
			A. braziliense (in cutaneous larva migrans)	
	Larvae voided in faeces Filariform, infective to new or same host Rhabditiform, metamorphose to filariform (infective)		Strongyloides stercoralis Direct cycle I Direct cycle II	5
(b) from WATER	Ova voided in urine or faeces HATCH in WATER to miracidia Penetrate SNAIL Develop to cercariae Liberated into WATER	Trematoda	Schistosoma haematobium	20
			S. mansoni	20
			S. japonicum	20
			Non-human schistosomes (in cercarial dermatitis)	
LARVAE INJECTED BY INSECTS (a) MOSQUITO spp	Microfilariae in blood or tissue juices ingested by insect	Nematoda	Wuchereria bancrofti	9
	MATURE in INSECT, now infective		Brugia malayi	10
(b) CHRYSOPS	Injected into man		Loa loa	11
(c) SIMULIUM			Onchocerca volvulus	12
			Dipetalonema perstans	10
(d) CULICOIDES spp	Pathogenicity to man doubtful		D. streptocerca	10
			Mansonella ozzardi	10

PLATE 30

ROUTES OF INFECTION Cont.

HUMAN INFECTION BY	ROUTE OUTSIDE BODY		CLASS	SPECIES	PLATE
ENCYSTED LARVAE EATEN					
(a) in CYCLOPS	Larvae from skin ulcer to WATER		Nematoda	Dracunculus medinensis	13
		Ingested by CYCLOPS			
		Encyst therein			
(b) in MEAT PORK	Larvae liberated in intestinal wall			Trichinella spiralis	7
		Encyst in flesh of SAME HOST			
	Ova voided in faeces	Ingested by PIGS	Cestoda	Taenia solium	14
		Encyst in flesh		(adult infection)	
BEEF		Ingested by CATTLE		Taenia saginata	15
		Encyst in flesh			
(c) in FRESHWATER FISH	Ova voided in faeces	MATURE IN WATER	Cestoda	Dibothriocephalus latus	17
		Hatch to coracidium			
		Ingested by CYCLOPS (etc)			
		Develop into procercoid			
		Cyclops ingested by FISH			
		Encyst in muscles plerocercoid (infective)			
		Ingested by SNAIL	Trematoda	Clonorchis sinensis	22
		Hatch in snail and develop to cercariae			
		Liberated to WATER			
		Penetrate cyprinoid FISH			
		Encyst as metacercariae (infective)			
(d) in CRUSTACEA	Ova voided in sputum or faeces	MATURE IN WATER		Paragonimus westermani	23
		Penetrate SNAIL			
		Development to cercariae			
		Liberated to WATER			
		Penetrate CRUSTACEANS			
		Encyst as metacercariae (infective)			
(e) on VEGETATION	Ova voided in faeces	MATURE IN SOIL		Fasciola hepatica	24
		Hatch to miracidia			
		Penetrate SNAIL		Fasciolopsis buski	25
		Development to cercariae			
		Liberated to VEGETATION			
		Encyst as metacercariae (infective)			
(f) in FLEAS	Ova voided in faeces	Ingested by FLEAS	Cestoda	Hymenolepis diminuta	16
		Develop into cysticercoid (infective)			

PART II
Protozoa of medical importance.

CONTENTS

PLATE

Abridged classification of Protozoa of Medical Importance ... 31
Basic Morphology of Protozoa ... 32
The Coccidia ... 33

The Malaria Parasite ... 34

Life Cycle of Malarial parasites *Plasmodium spp:* ... 35
Morphology of Malarial parasites ... 36
Morphology of Malarial parasites (*cont.*) ... 37
Morphology of Malarial parasites (*cont.*) ... 38
Morphology of Malarial parasites (*cont.*) ... 39
Morphology in stained thick films ... 40
Pigment in oocysts ... 41
The Pathogenesis of Malaria ... 42
Pathology of Malaria: 1. Acute phase ... 43
2. Chronic phase ... 44
3. Complications and sequelae ... 45
4. Black water fever ... 46
Laboratory Diagnosis of Malaria ... 47

Sarcocystis lindemanni ... 48

The Amoebae of the Intestinal Canal ... 49

Life cycle of *Entamoeba histolytica* ... 50
Entamoeba histolytica : morphology ... 51
Entamoeba histolytica : morphology (*cont.*) ... 52
Amoebiasis: Pathology ... 53
Amoebiasis: Pathology (*cont.*) ... 54
Laboratory Diagnosis of Amoebiasis ... 55
The Non-Pathogenic Intestinal Amoebae ... 56

Entamoeba coli
Endolimax nana
Iodamoeba bütschlii
Dientamoeba fragilis

The Body Fluid or Tissue Flagellates ... 57

Classification and morphology of *Leishmania spp.* ... 57
Leishmaniasis: Life cycle ... 58
Visceral Leishmaniasis ... 59
Cutaneous Leishmaniasis ... 60
Mucocutaneous Leishmaniasis ... 60
Diagnosis of Leishmaniasis ... 60
African Trypanosomiasis ... 61
Life cycle of *T. gambiense* and *T. rhodesiense* ... 61
Pathology ... 62
Diagnosis ... 65
South American Trypanosomiasis ... 63
Life cycle of *T. Cruzi* ... 63
Pathology ... 64
Diagnosis ... 65
Morphology of human and animal trypanosomes ... 67

Recapitulation: Difference Between Trypanosomiasis and Visceral Leishmaniasis ... 66

The Intestinal Flagellates ... 68

Giardia lamblia
Chilomastix mesnili
Trichomonas spp.

The Ciliata—*Balantidium coli* ... 69
Protozoa of uncertain status : *Toxoplasma gondii* and *Pneumocystis carinii* ... 70
Recapitulation: Tissue protozoa ... 71
Intestinal protozoa

Abridged classification of Protozoa of Medical Importance

PHYLUM — PROTOZOA (UNICELLULAR ORGANISMS)

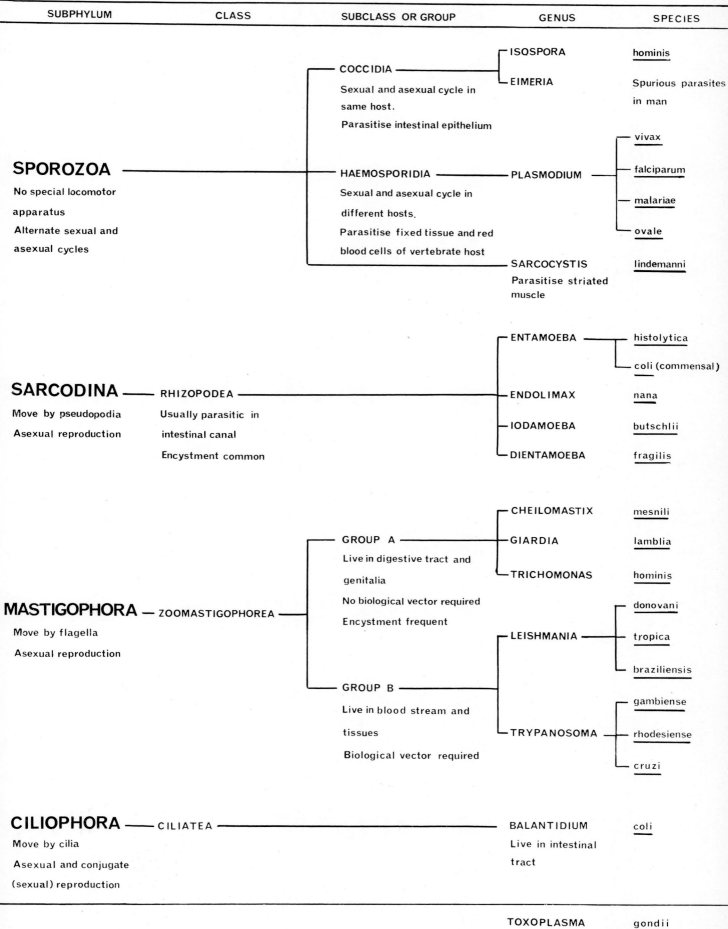

SUBPHYLUM	CLASS	SUBCLASS OR GROUP	GENUS	SPECIES
SPOROZOA — No special locomotor apparatus. Alternate sexual and asexual cycles		COCCIDIA — Sexual and asexual cycle in same host. Parasitise intestinal epithelium	ISOSPORA	hominis
			EIMERIA	Spurious parasites in man
		HAEMOSPORIDIA — Sexual and asexual cycle in different hosts. Parasitise fixed tissue and red blood cells of vertebrate host	PLASMODIUM	vivax / falciparum / malariae / ovale
			SARCOCYSTIS — Parasitise striated muscle	lindemanni
SARCODINA — Move by pseudopodia. Asexual reproduction	RHIZOPODEA — Usually parasitic in intestinal canal. Encystment common		ENTAMOEBA	histolytica / coli (commensal)
			ENDOLIMAX	nana
			IODAMOEBA	butschlii
			DIENTAMOEBA	fragilis
MASTIGOPHORA — Move by flagella. Asexual reproduction	ZOOMASTIGOPHOREA	GROUP A — Live in digestive tract and genitalia. No biological vector required. Encystment frequent	CHEILOMASTIX	mesnili
			GIARDIA	lamblia
			TRICHOMONAS	hominis
		GROUP B — Live in blood stream and tissues. Biological vector required	LEISHMANIA	donovani / tropica / braziliensis
			TRYPANOSOMA	gambiense / rhodesiense / cruzi
CILIOPHORA — Move by cilia. Asexual and conjugate (sexual) reproduction	CILIATEA		BALANTIDIUM — Live in intestinal tract	coli

OF UNCERTAIN STATUS — No special locomotor apparatus. No sexual stage

| | | | TOXOPLASMA — Parasitic in various organs | gondii |
| PNEUMOCYSTIS — Parasitic in respiratory passages | carinii |

PLATE 32

Basic morphology of Protozoa

LOCOMOTOR APPARATUS

NO SPECIAL

PSEUDOPODIA

FLAGELLA

PARABASAL BODY
BLEPHAROPLAST
AXONEME
KINETOPLAST

Sometimes connected to body by undulating membrane

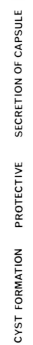

CILIA

ADAPTATION FOR SURVIVAL

DIRECT HOST TO HOST TRANSFER OF TROPHIC STAGE

CYST FORMATION   PROTECTIVE   SECRETION OF CAPSULE

REPRODUCTIVE   nucleus divides

often food store
(chromidial bars)

HOST TO HOST TRANSFER via INTERMEDIATE HOST
(usually invertebrate)

SEXUAL STAGES IN LIFE CYCLE

1 NUCLEUS

May be single or multiple

FOR LIFE, REPRODUCTION. GENETIC TRANSMISSION

Nuclear membrane

Nucleoplasm

Chromatin   Compact

Scattered sometimes with –Karyosome

Important in recognition
of *Rhizopoda*

Particles throughout

Lining nuclear membrane

2 ENDOPLASM

Moderately dense–granular

FOR FOOD SYNTHESIS

Food storage in vacuoles (undigested)

As chromidial bars (glycogen or protein)

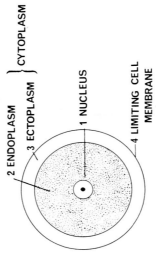

2 ENDOPLASM
3 ECTOPLASM
1 NUCLEUS
4 LIMITING CELL MEMBRANE
CYTOPLASM

3 ECTOPLASM

Homogeneous

FOR PROCUREMENT AND INGESTION OF FOOD   Absorbed anywhere

Specialised cell mouth (cytostome)

Predigested

Digestion of host tissue

FOR RESPIRATION Aerobic or anaerobic

FOR DISCHARGE WASTE PRODUCTS   At any site

May collect in vacuoles first

May have specialised cell anus

FOR PROTECTION

May have contractile vacuoles (in *Balantidium coli*)

4 LIMITING CELL MEMBRANE

May have ⌐ no constant shape
⌐ more or less constant shape

The Coccidia

PLATE 33

Classification

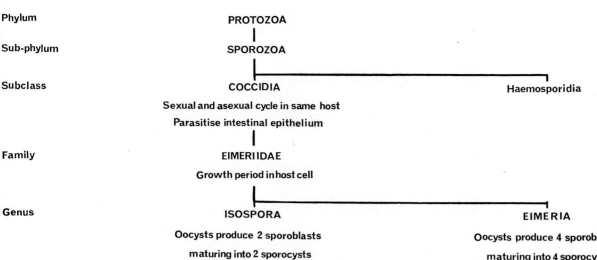

Phylum	PROTOZOA	
Sub-phylum	SPOROZOA	
Subclass	COCCIDIA	Haemosporidia

COCCIDIA
Sexual and asexual cycle in same host
Parasitise intestinal epithelium

Family	EIMERIIDAE

Growth period in host cell

Genus	ISOSPORA	EIMERIA

ISOSPORA
Oocysts produce 2 sporoblasts
maturing into 2 sporocysts
each developing 4 sporozoites

EIMERIA
Oocysts produce 4 sporoblasts
maturing into 4 sporocysts
each developing 2 sporozoites

Oocyst Morphology

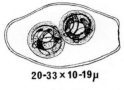

20-33 × 10-19μ

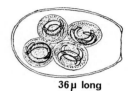

36μ long

Species

I. belli
I. hominis

Spurious parasites in man from eating
infected fish. Only important re differentiation
of oocysts in faeces.

ISOSPORA
(Causing Coccidiosis in man)

MORPHOLOGY   Apart from oocyst (above) unknown in man.

Life cycle   (Conjectural, based on animal data.)

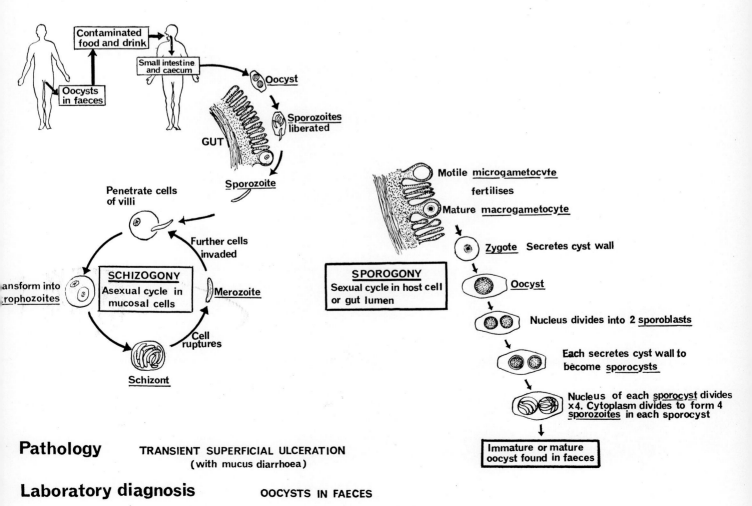

Contaminated food and drink

Small intestine and caecum

Oocysts in faeces

Oocyst

Sporozoites liberated

GUT

Sporozoite

Penetrate cells of villi

Further cells invaded

transform into trophozoites

SCHIZOGONY
Asexual cycle in mucosal cells

Merozoite

Cell ruptures

Schizont

Motile microgametocyte
fertilises
Mature macrogametocyte

Zygote   Secretes cyst wall

SPOROGONY
Sexual cycle in host cell or gut lumen

Oocyst

Nucleus divides into 2 sporoblasts

Each secretes cyst wall to become sporocysts

Nucleus of each sporocyst divides × 4. Cytoplasm divides to form 4 sporozoites in each sporocyst

Immature or mature oocyst found in faeces

Pathology   TRANSIENT SUPERFICIAL ULCERATION
(with mucus diarrhoea)

Laboratory diagnosis   OOCYSTS IN FAECES

The Malarial Parasite

PLATE 34

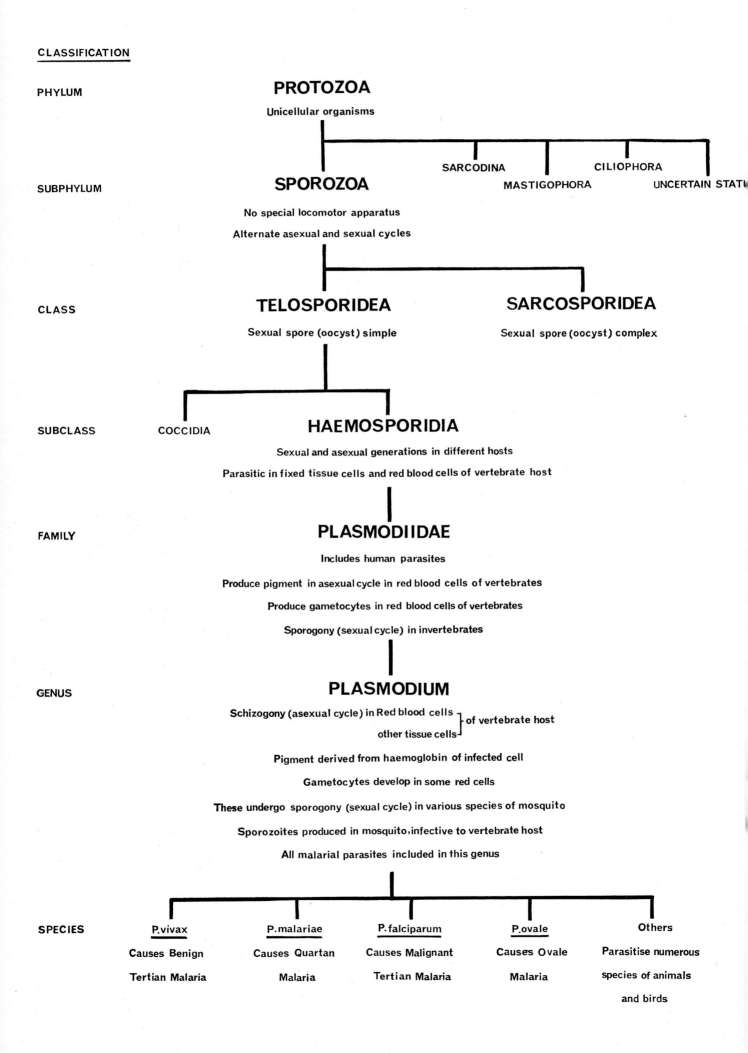

CLASSIFICATION

PHYLUM

PROTOZOA

Unicellular organisms

SUBPHYLUM

SPOROZOA   SARCODINA   CILIOPHORA

MASTIGOPHORA   UNCERTAIN STATU

No special locomotor apparatus

Alternate asexual and sexual cycles

CLASS

TELOSPORIDEA   **SARCOSPORIDEA**

Sexual spore (oocyst) simple   Sexual spore (oocyst) complex

SUBCLASS   COCCIDIA   **HAEMOSPORIDIA**

Sexual and asexual generations in different hosts

Parasitic in fixed tissue cells and red blood cells of vertebrate host

FAMILY

PLASMODIIDAE

Includes human parasites

Produce pigment in asexual cycle in red blood cells of vertebrates

Produce gametocytes in red blood cells of vertebrates

Sporogony (sexual cycle) in invertebrates

GENUS

PLASMODIUM

Schizogony (asexual cycle) in Red blood cells
other tissue cells — of vertebrate host

Pigment derived from haemoglobin of infected cell

Gametocytes develop in some red cells

These undergo sporogony (sexual cycle) in various species of mosquito

Sporozoites produced in mosquito, infective to vertebrate host

All malarial parasites included in this genus

SPECIES	P.vivax	P.malariae	P.falciparum	P.ovale	Others
	Causes Benign	Causes Quartan	Causes Malignant	Causes Ovale	Parasitise numerous
	Tertian Malaria	Malaria	Tertian Malaria	Malaria	species of animals
					and birds

PLATE 35

Life cycle of Malarial parasites.

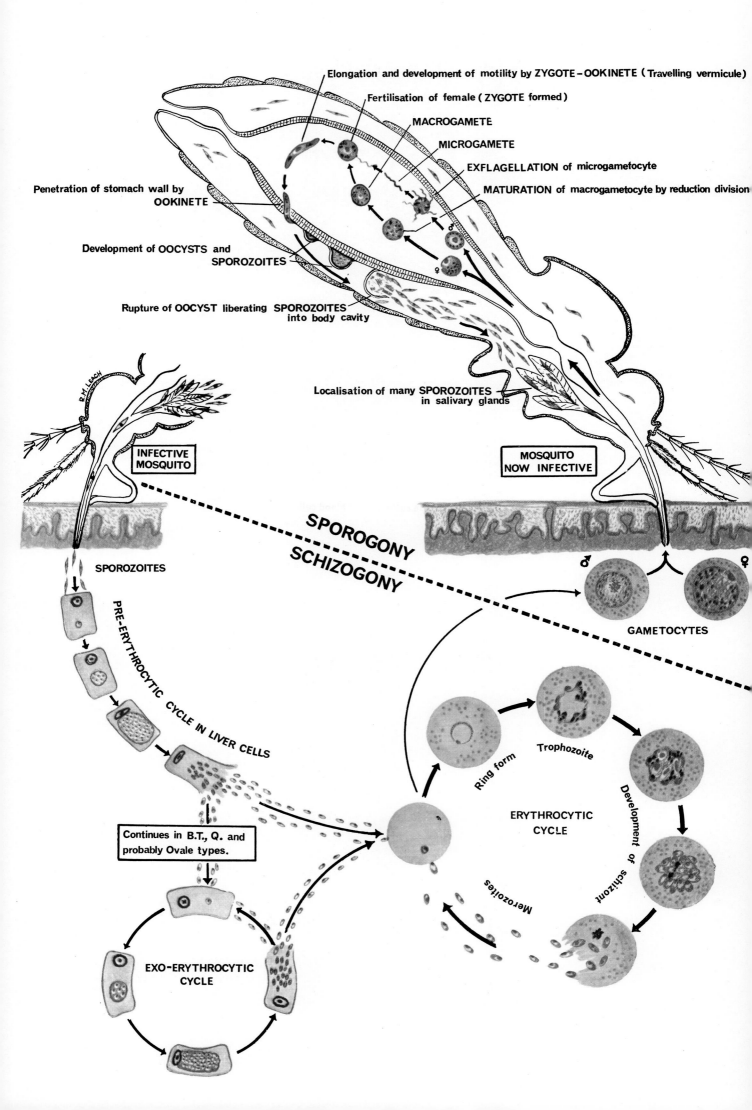

Elongation and development of motility by ZYGOTE – OOKINETE (Travelling vermicule)

Fertilisation of female (ZYGOTE formed)

MACROGAMETE

MICROGAMETE

EXFLAGELLATION of microgametocyte

MATURATION of macrogametocyte by reduction division

Penetration of stomach wall by OOKINETE

Development of OOCYSTS and SPOROZOITES

Rupture of OOCYST liberating SPOROZOITES into body cavity

Localisation of many SPOROZOITES in salivary glands

R.M.LEACH

INFECTIVE MOSQUITO

MOSQUITO NOW INFECTIVE

SPOROGONY

SCHIZOGONY

GAMETOCYTES

SPOROZOITES

PRE-ERYTHROCYTIC CYCLE IN LIVER CELLS

Continues in B.T., Q. and probably Ovale types.

EXO-ERYTHROCYTIC CYCLE

Ring form

Trophozoite

ERYTHROCYTIC CYCLE

Development of schizont

Merozoites

PLATE 36

Morphology of Malarial parasites.

Stained by Leishman or Giemsa

SCHIZOGONY (Asexual cycle)

EXO-ERYTHROCYTIC CYCLE IN LIVER CELLS

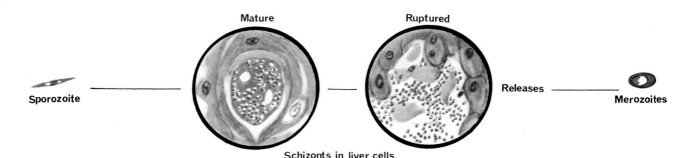

Sporozoite

Mature

Ruptured

Releases

Merozoites

Schizonts in liver cells

NO PIGMENT AT THIS STAGE

NO SURROUNDING REACTION

ERYTHROCYTIC STAGE IN RED CELLS

General features

CYTOPLASM BLUE

CHROMATIN RED

The parasite

PIGMENT (from haemoglobin) varies in colour

time of appearance

The red cell

SIZE

Normal

MAY VARY IN

SHAPE

R B C

MAY CONTAIN

SCHUFFNER'S
DOTS

Pink spots in cytoplasm
unoccupied by parasite

MAURER'S
CLEFTS

Brick red clefts
in cytoplasm

	P. vivax	P. malariae	P. falciparum	P. ovale
SIZE	ENLARGED	NOT ENLARGED	NOT ENLARGED	SLIGHTLY ENLARGED
COLOUR	PALE	NORMAL	NORMAL	PALE
SHAPE	ROUND	ROUND	ROUND MAY BE CRENATED	OVAL MAY BE FIMBRIATED
SCHUFFNER'S DOTS	PRESENT	NONE	NONE	CONSPICUOUS
MAURER'S CLEFTS	NONE	NONE	MAY BE PRESENT	NONE

Morphology of Malaria parasites

PLATE 37

STAGES IN THIN FILMS

P. vivax	P. malariae	P. falciparum	P. ovale

RING FORMS (EARLY TROPHOZOITES)

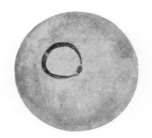 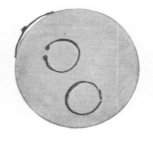 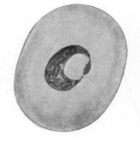

	P. vivax	P. malariae	P. falciparum	P. ovale
SIZE	⅓ RED CELL	UP TO ⅓	⅕ RED CELL	⅓ RED CELL
SHAPE	DELICATE RING	COMPACT RING	VERY DELICATE RING	DENSE RING
CHROMATIN	FINE DOT SOMETIMES TWO	ONE MASS OFTEN INSIDE RING	FINE DOTS FREQUENTLY TWO	DENSE, WELL DEFINED MASS
ACCOLÉ FORMS	SOMETIMES	NONE	FREQUENT	NONE
PIGMENT	NONE AT THIS STAGE	MAY BE PRESENT	NONE AT THIS STAGE	NONE AT THIS STAGE

DEVELOPING TROPHOZOITES

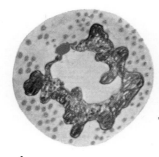 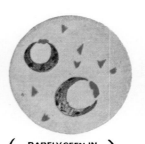 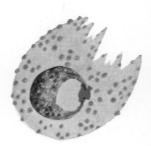

(RARELY SEEN IN PERIPHERAL BLOOD)

	P. vivax	P. malariae	P. falciparum	P. ovale
SIZE	LARGE	SMALL	SMALL	SMALL
SHAPE	VERY IRREGULAR	COMPACT, OFTEN BAND FORMS	COMPACT	COMPACT
VACUOLE	PROMINENT	INCONSPICUOUS	INCONSPICUOUS	INCONSPICUOUS
CHROMATIN	DOTS OR THREADS	DOTS OR THREADS	DOTS OR THREADS	LARGE IRREGULAR CLUMPS
PIGMENT TEXTURE	FINE	COARSE	COARSE	COARSE
COLOUR	YELLOW BROWN	DARK BROWN	BLACK	DARK YELLOW BROWN
QUANTITY	MEDIUM	ABUNDANT	MEDIUM	MEDIUM
DISTRIBUTION	SCATTERED FINE PARTICLES	SCATTERED CLUMPS AND RODS	AGGREGATED IN TWO CLUMPS	SCATTERED COARSE PARTICLES

PLATE 38

Morphology of Malaria parasites (cont.)

	P.vivax	**P.malariae**	**P.falciparum**	**P.ovale**

IMMATURE SCHIZONTS

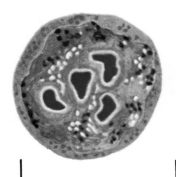 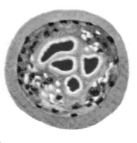 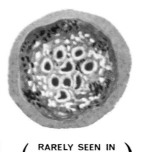 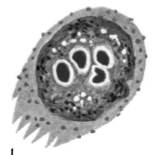

	P.vivax	**P.malariae**	**P.falciparum** (RARELY SEEN IN PERIPHERAL BLOOD)	**P.ovale**
SIZE	ALMOST FILLS RED CELL	ALMOST FILLS RED CELL	ALMOST FILLS RED CELL	ALMOST FILLS RED CELL
SHAPE	SOMEWHAT AMOEBOID	COMPACT	COMPACT	COMPACT
CHROMATIN	NUMEROUS IRREGULAR MASSES	FEW IRREGULAR MASSES	NUMEROUS IRREGULAR MASSES	FEW IRREGULAR MASSES
PIGMENT	SCATTERED	SCATTERED	SCATTERED	SCATTERED

MATURE SCHIZONTS

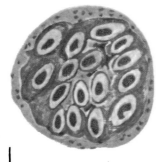 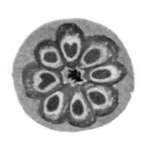 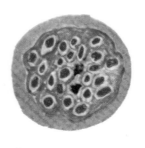 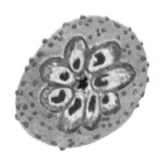

		P.vivax	**P.malariae**	**P.falciparum** (RARELY SEEN IN PERIPHERAL BLOOD)	**P.ovale**
SIZE		FILLS RED CELL	NEARLY FILLS RED CELL	NEARLY FILLS RED CELL	FILLS ¾ OF RED CELL
SHAPE		SEGMENTED	SEGMENTED DAISY HEAD	SEGMENTED	SEGMENTED
MEROZOITES	RANGE	14 — 24	6 — 12	8 — 32	6 — 12
	MEAN	16	8	24	8
	SIZE	MEDIUM	LARGE	SMALL	LARGE
PIGMENT		AGGREGATED IN CENTRE (YELLOW BROWN)	AGGREGATED IN CENTRE (DARK BROWN)	AGGREGATED IN CENTRE (BLACK)	AGGREGATED IN CENTRE (DARK YELLOW BROWN)

PLATE 39

Morphology of Malaria parasites (cont.)

MICROGAMETOCYTES

	P.vivax	P.malariae	P.falciparum	P.ovale
	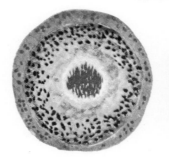	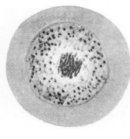	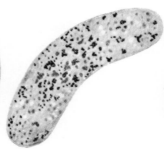	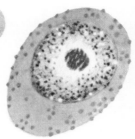
TIME OF APPEARANCE	3–5 DAYS	7–14 DAYS	7–12 DAYS	12–14 DAYS
NUMBER IN BLOOD STREAM	MANY	SCANTY	MANY	SCANTY
SIZE	FILLS ENLARGED RED CELL	SMALLER THAN RED CELL	LARGER THAN RED CELL	SIZE OF RED CELL
SHAPE	ROUND OR OVAL COMPACT	ROUND COMPACT	KIDNEY SHAPED BLUNTLY ROUND ENDS	ROUND COMPACT
CYTOPLASM	PALE BLUE	PALE BLUE	REDDISH BLUE	PALE BLUE
CHROMATIN	FIBRILS IN SKEIN WITH SURROUNDING UNSTAINED AREA	AS FOR P.vivax	FINE GRANULES SCATTERED THROUGHOUT	AS FOR P.vivax
PIGMENT	ABUNDANT BROWN GRANULES THROUGHOUT	AS FOR P.vivax	DARK GRANULES THROUGHOUT	AS FOR P.vivax

MACROGAMETOCYTES

	P.vivax	P.malariae	P.falciparum	P.ovale
	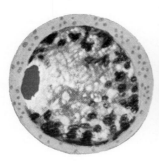	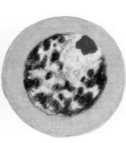	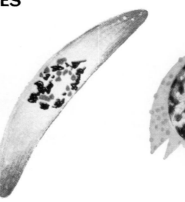	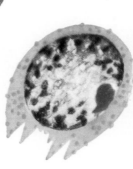
TIME OF APPEARANCE	3–5 DAYS	7–14 DAYS	7–12 DAYS	12–14 DAYS
NUMBER IN BLOOD STREAM	MANY	SCANTY	MANY	SCANTY
SIZE	FILLS ENLARGED RED CELL	SMALLER THAN RED CELL	LARGER THAN RED CELL	SIZE OF RED CELL
SHAPE	ROUND OR OVAL COMPACT	ROUND COMPACT	CRESCENTIC–SHARPLY ROUNDED OR POINTED ENDS	ROUND COMPACT
CYTOPLASM	DARK BLUE	DARK BLUE	DARK BLUE	DARK BLUE
CHROMATIN	COMPACT PERIPHERAL MASS	AS FOR P.vivax	COMPACT MASSES NEAR CENTRE	AS FOR P.vivax
PIGMENT	SMALL MASSES ROUND PERIPHERY	AS FOR P.vivax	BLACK GRANULES ROUND NUCLEUS	AS FOR P.vivax

Morphology in stained thick films

PLATE 40

GENERAL

PARASITES NOT FLATTENED SO ARE SMALLER THAN IN THIN FILM

RED CELLS HAEMOLYSED IN PROCESSING SO NO GUIDE TO :- SIZE
SHAPE } OF RED BLOOD CELL
COLOUR

SCHUFFNER'S DOTS INDEFINITE   NO MAURER'S CLEFTS.

PARTICULAR

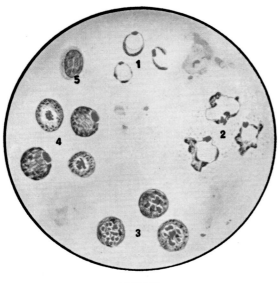

P. vivax

1. RING FORMS. SMALL FINE RINGS OFTEN BROKEN

2. TROPHOZOITES. MARKEDLY IRREGULAR CYTOPLASM

3. SCHIZONTS. MANY (AVERAGE 16) SMALL MEROZOITES

4. GAMETOCYTES. COMPACT PARASITES WITH FEATURES OF
♂ AND ♀. AS DESCRIBED

5. WHITE BLOOD CELL

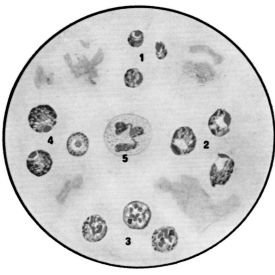

P. malariae
P. ovale } ALMOST IDENTICAL BUT SCHÜFFNER'S DOTS MAY BE VISIBLE IN LATTER

1. RING FORMS. COMPACT RINGS

2. TROPHOZOITES. SOLID REGULAR CYTOPLASM

3. SCHIZONTS. FEW (AVERAGE 8) LARGE MEROZOITES

4. GAMETOCYTES. VERY DIFFICULT TO DISTINGUISH
FROM P. VIVAX

5. WHITE BLOOD CELL

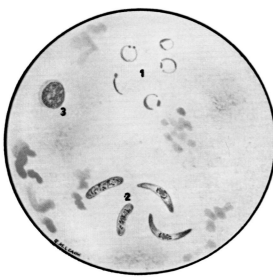

P. falciparum

1. RING FORMS. VERY SMALL, FINE RINGS USUALLY UNBROKEN

TROPHOZOITES }
} NOT SEEN IN PERIPHERAL BLOOD USUALLY
SCHIZONTS }

2. GAMETOCYTES. CHARACTERISTIC CRESCENTIC ♂ AND ♀ FORMS

3. WHITE BLOOD CELL

PLATE 41

Malaria

SPECIES IDENTIFICATION IN THE MOSQUITO – PIGMENT IN OOCYSTS

Oocysts	P. vivax	P. malariae	P. falciparum	P. ovale
LENGTH OF CYCLE IN DAYS	9	15–21	10	15
SIZE IN μ	10–46	5–44	8–60	9–37
PIGMENT COLOUR	Greenish brown	Dark brown or nearly black	Blackish	Dark brown or nearly black
TEXTURE	Fine	Medium coarse	Very coarse	Medium coarse
NUMBER OF GRAINS	50–100	30	10–20	50–60

PATTERN

DAYS

3 — None

4, 5 — Typical Prince of Wales feather design

P. malariae: Distributed, some clumping

6 — P. falciparum: Concentrated at periphery in double row often

P. ovale: Concentrated at periphery in semi-circles or dotted lines

7, 8, 9, 10 — P. vivax: Obscured by nuclei

P. malariae: Increased clumping

P. falciparum: Mainly obscured

P. ovale: Most clearly defined, dotted lines often crossed

After 10 — P. malariae: If visible, clumped at periphery

P. falciparum: Seldom visible

P. ovale: Mainly obscured

RECAPITULATION OF DISTINCTIVE FEATURES

P. vivax: Prince of Wales feather design

P. malariae: Distributed then clumped

P. falciparum: Peripheral in rows

P. ovale: Semicircular or crossed line design

(Adapted from Shute)

PLATE 42

The Pathogenesis of Malaria

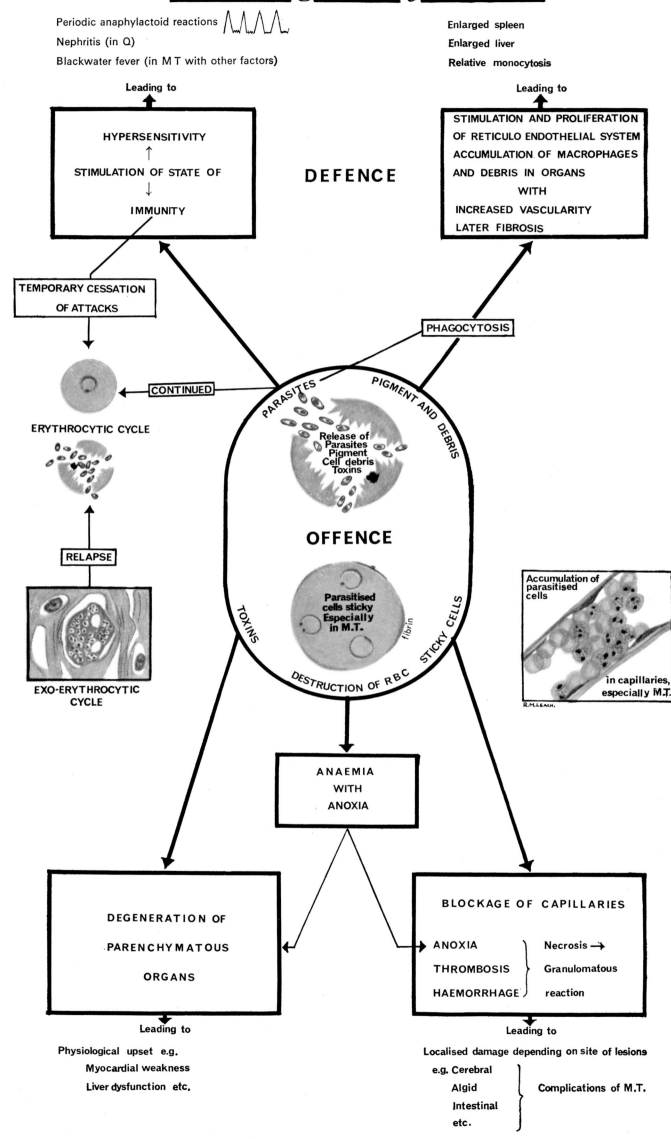

Periodic anaphylactoid reactions

Nephritis (in Q)

Blackwater fever (in M T with other factors)

Enlarged spleen

Enlarged liver

Relative monocytosis

Leading to

Leading to

HYPERSENSITIVITY
↑
STIMULATION OF STATE OF
↓
IMMUNITY

DEFENCE

STIMULATION AND PROLIFERATION
OF RETICULO ENDOTHELIAL SYSTEM
ACCUMULATION OF MACROPHAGES
AND DEBRIS IN ORGANS
WITH
INCREASED VASCULARITY
LATER FIBROSIS

TEMPORARY CESSATION
OF ATTACKS

PHAGOCYTOSIS

CONTINUED

ERYTHROCYTIC CYCLE

PARASITES

PIGMENT AND DEBRIS

Release of
Parasites
Pigment
Cell debris
Toxins

RELAPSE

OFFENCE

EXO-ERYTHROCYTIC
CYCLE

TOXINS

Parasitised
cells sticky
Especially
in M.T.

fibrin

DESTRUCTION OF RBC   STICKY CELLS

Accumulation of
parasitised
cells

in capillaries,
especially M.T.

R.M.LEACH.

ANAEMIA
WITH
ANOXIA

DEGENERATION OF

PARENCHYMATOUS

ORGANS

BLOCKAGE OF CAPILLARIES

ANOXIA   Necrosis →

THROMBOSIS   Granulomatous

HAEMORRHAGE   reaction

Leading to

Physiological upset e.g.
Myocardial weakness
Liver dysfunction etc.

Leading to

Localised damage depending on site of lesions
e.g. Cerebral
Algid   Complications of M.T.
Intestinal
etc.

PLATE 43

Pathology of Malaria

(1) ACUTE PHASE

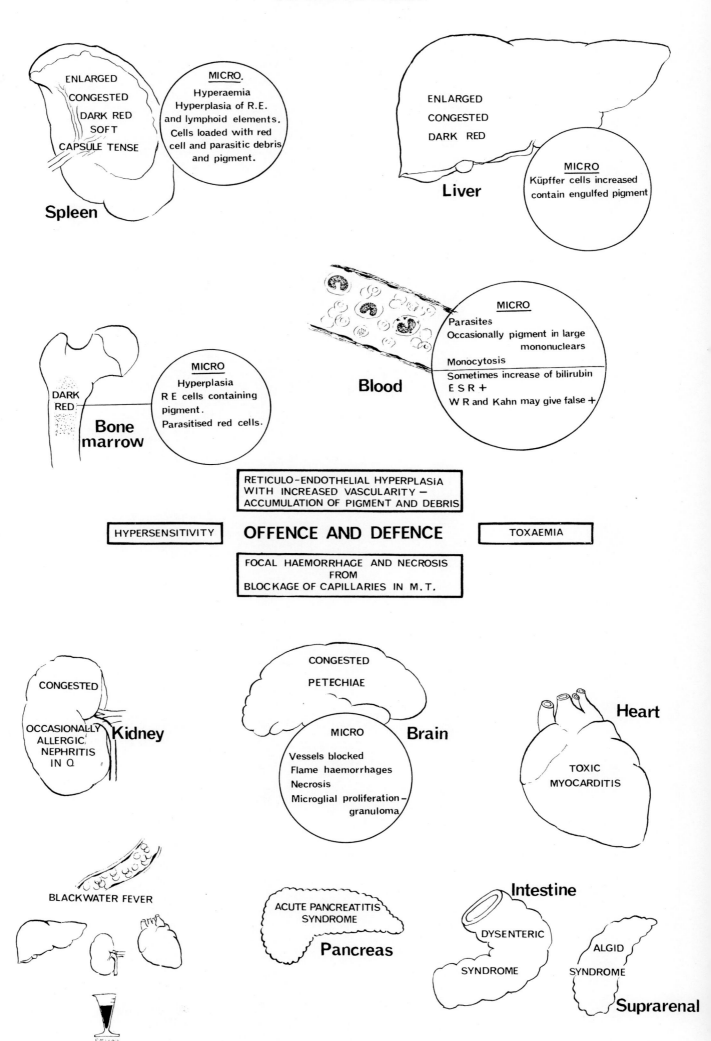

Spleen
ENLARGED
CONGESTED
DARK RED
SOFT
CAPSULE TENSE

MICRO.
Hyperaemia
Hyperplasia of R.E.
and lymphoid elements.
Cells loaded with red
cell and parasitic debris
and pigment.

Liver
ENLARGED
CONGESTED
DARK RED

MICRO
Küpffer cells increased
contain engulfed pigment

Bone marrow
DARK RED

MICRO
Hyperplasia
R E cells containing
pigment.
Parasitised red cells.

Blood
MICRO
Parasites
Occasionally pigment in large
mononuclears
Monocytosis
Sometimes increase of bilirubin
E S R +
W R and Kahn may give false +

RETICULO-ENDOTHELIAL HYPERPLASIA
WITH INCREASED VASCULARITY —
ACCUMULATION OF PIGMENT AND DEBRIS

HYPERSENSITIVITY

OFFENCE AND DEFENCE

TOXAEMIA

FOCAL HAEMORRHAGE AND NECROSIS
FROM
BLOCKAGE OF CAPILLARIES IN M.T.

Kidney
CONGESTED
OCCASIONALLY
ALLERGIC
NEPHRITIS
IN Q

Brain
CONGESTED
PETECHIAE

MICRO
Vessels blocked
Flame haemorrhages
Necrosis
Microglial proliferation —
granuloma

Heart
TOXIC
MYOCARDITIS

BLACKWATER FEVER

ACUTE PANCREATITIS
SYNDROME
Pancreas

Intestine
DYSENTERIC
SYNDROME

ALGID
SYNDROME
Suprarenal

PLATE 44

Pathology of Malaria

(2) CHRONIC PHASE

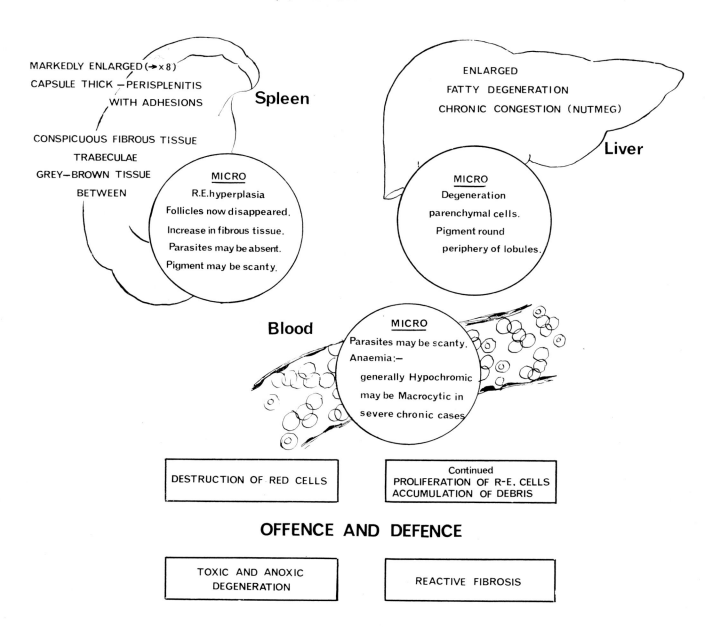

Spleen

MARKEDLY ENLARGED (→ x 8)

CAPSULE THICK — PERISPLENITIS

WITH ADHESIONS

CONSPICUOUS FIBROUS TISSUE

TRABECULAE

GREY—BROWN TISSUE

BETWEEN

MICRO
R.E. hyperplasia
Follicles now disappeared.
Increase in fibrous tissue.
Parasites may be absent.
Pigment may be scanty.

Liver

ENLARGED

FATTY DEGENERATION

CHRONIC CONGESTION (NUTMEG)

MICRO
Degeneration
parenchymal cells.
Pigment round
periphery of lobules.

Blood

MICRO
Parasites may be scanty.
Anaemia:—
generally Hypochromic
may be Macrocytic in
severe chronic cases

DESTRUCTION OF RED CELLS

Continued
PROLIFERATION OF R-E. CELLS
ACCUMULATION OF DEBRIS

OFFENCE AND DEFENCE

TOXIC AND ANOXIC
DEGENERATION

REACTIVE FIBROSIS

Heart

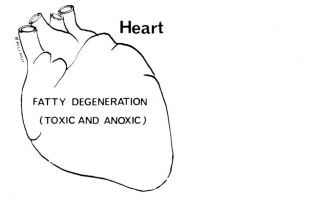

FATTY DEGENERATION
(TOXIC AND ANOXIC)

Bone marrow

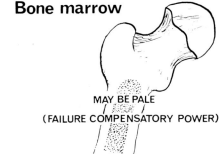

MAY BE PALE
(FAILURE COMPENSATORY POWER)

PLATE 45

Pathology of Malaria

(3) COMPLICATIONS AND SEQUELAE

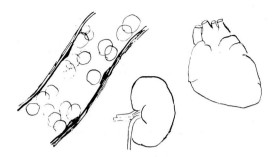

BLACKWATER FEVER
(See PLATE 46)

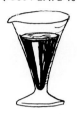

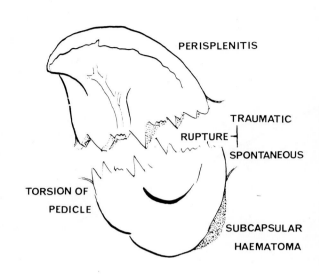

PERISPLENITIS

TRAUMATIC

RUPTURE

SPONTANEOUS

TORSION OF
PEDICLE

SUBCAPSULAR
HAEMATOMA

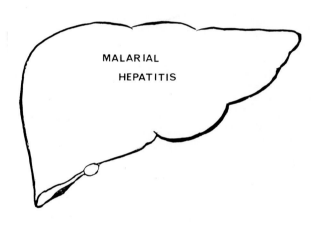

MALARIAL
HEPATITIS

NEURALGIA   RETINAL HAEMORRHAGES

INTERSTITIAL   CATARACT
KERATITIS

OCULAR (RARE)

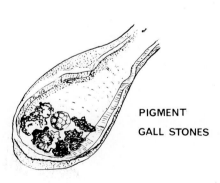

PIGMENT
GALL STONES

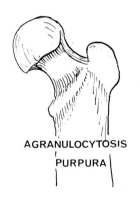

AGRANULOCYTOSIS
PURPURA

ANAEMIA ⟶ **Decreased General Resistance** ⟶ INTERCURRENT DISEASE
DEBILITY

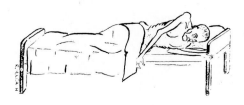

PLATE 46

Pathology of Malaria

(4) BLACKWATER FEVER

(SEE PLATE 45)

ACUTE HAEMOLYTIC ATTACKS IN M.T. MALARIA ; ASSOCIATED WITH TAKING OF QUININE ; NUMEROUS THEORIES AS TO MECHANISM

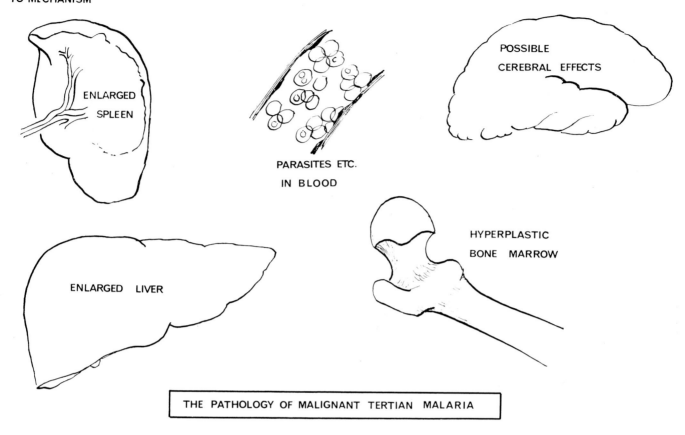

POSSIBLE CEREBRAL EFFECTS

ENLARGED SPLEEN

PARASITES ETC. IN BLOOD

ENLARGED LIVER

HYPERPLASTIC BONE MARROW

THE PATHOLOGY OF MALIGNANT TERTIAN MALARIA

OFFENCE AND DEFENCE

PLUS

ATTACK(S) OF MASSIVE INTRAVASCULAR HAEMOLYSIS

WITH

ACUTE ANOXIA

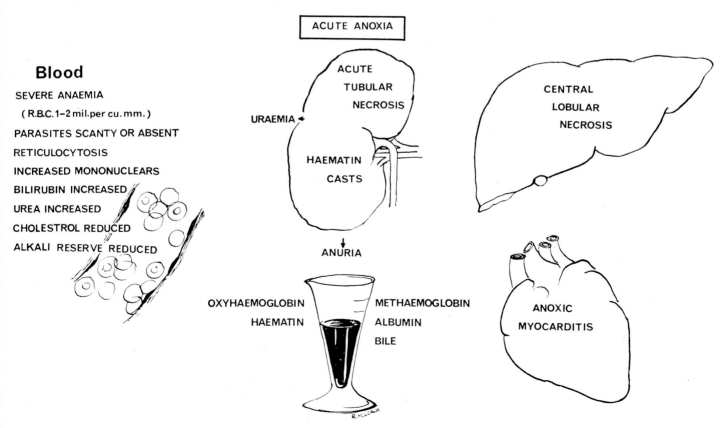

Blood

SEVERE ANAEMIA

(R.B.C. 1–2 mil. per cu. mm.)

PARASITES SCANTY OR ABSENT

RETICULOCYTOSIS

INCREASED MONONUCLEARS

BILIRUBIN INCREASED

UREA INCREASED

CHOLESTROL REDUCED

ALKALI RESERVE REDUCED

ACUTE TUBULAR NECROSIS

URAEMIA

HAEMATIN CASTS

CENTRAL LOBULAR NECROSIS

ANURIA

OXYHAEMOGLOBIN
HAEMATIN

METHAEMOGLOBIN
ALBUMIN
BILE

ANOXIC MYOCARDITIS

Laboratory Diagnosis of Malaria

PLATE 47

Malarial parasites in thin film of blood. Stained by Leishman and Giemsa

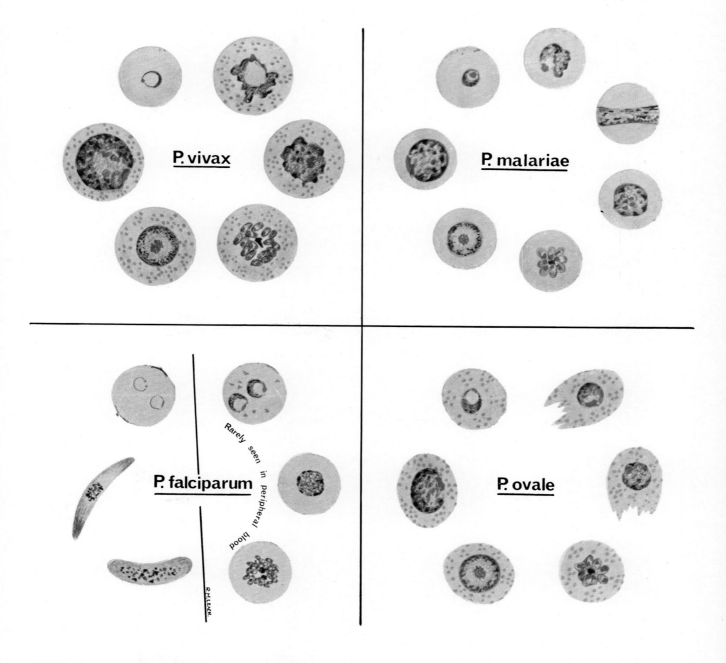

P. vivax

P. malariae

P. falciparum

Rarely seen in peripheral blood

P. ovale

THICK FILM OF BLOOD STAINED BY FIELD OR GIEMSA

IN THICK OR THIN FILM OF BONE MARROW

CONCENTRATION

SEROLOGICAL   } TECHNIQUES ACADEMIC RATHER THAN PRACTICAL

CULTURAL

BLACK WATER FEVER

IN ADDITION TO ABOVE

SPECTROSCOPIC EXAMINATION OF URINE AND FAECES

TESTS TO EXCLUDE OTHER CAUSES OF HAEMOGLOBINURIA

(e.g. Donäth-Landsteiner reaction for cold agglutinins.)

PLATE 48

Sarcocystis lindemanni

CLASSIFICATION

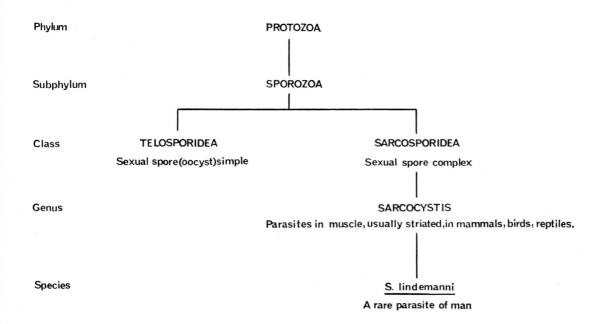

Phylum	PROTOZOA	
Subphylum	SPOROZOA	
Class	TELOSPORIDEA Sexual spore(oocyst)simple	SARCOSPORIDEA Sexual spore complex
Genus		SARCOCYSTIS Parasites in muscle, usually striated, in mammals, birds, reptiles.
Species		S. lindemanni A rare parasite of man

PROBABLE LIFE CYCLE

(Based on animal data)

Cyst in muscle or excreta of infected animal — ingested — spores freed — enter intestinal epithelium — multiply — migrate to muscular tissue-grow into other cysts

MORPHOLOGY

Cyst in muscle only known

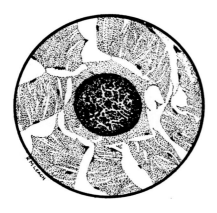

Cyst in human muscle
Miescher's tube ×100

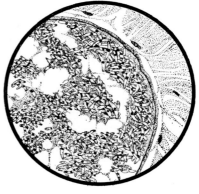

Enlarged portion of Miescher's tube showing Rainey's corpuscles (each 12–16×4–9 μ): from a human case

PATHOLOGY

Slight in man

Allergy – eosinophilia

Muscular swellings

LABORATORY DIAGNOSIS

Histology of biopsy specimen

PLATE 49

The Amoebae of The Intestinal Canal

Classification

Phylum   **Protozoa**

Sub phylum   **Sarcodina**   Sporozoa   Mastigophora   Ciliophora   Uncertain status

Move by pseudopodia

Asexual reproduction by binary fission

Class   **Rhizopoda**

Encystment common

Usually parasitise intestinal canal

Genera primarily differentiated by nuclear structure

Genera   **Entamoeba**

Generally one nucleus in trophozoite

Small karyosome at or near centre

Nuclear membrane lined with chromatin granules

Forms cysts

Endolimax

Generally one nucleus in trophozoite

Large irregular karyosome attached

to nuclear membrane

No peripheral chromatin

Forms cysts

Iodamoeba

Generally one nucleus in trophozoite

Large karyosome surrounded by achromatic granules

No peripheral chromatin

Forms cysts

Dientamoeba

Minute

Generally binucleate

Central particulate karyosome

No peripheral chromatin

No cystic stage

Species   **E. histolytica**   **E. nana**   **I. butschlii**   **D. fragilis**

E. coli

Entamoeba histolytica.
(Causing AMOEBIASIS)
LIFE CYCLE

PLATE 50

1 Inside the host

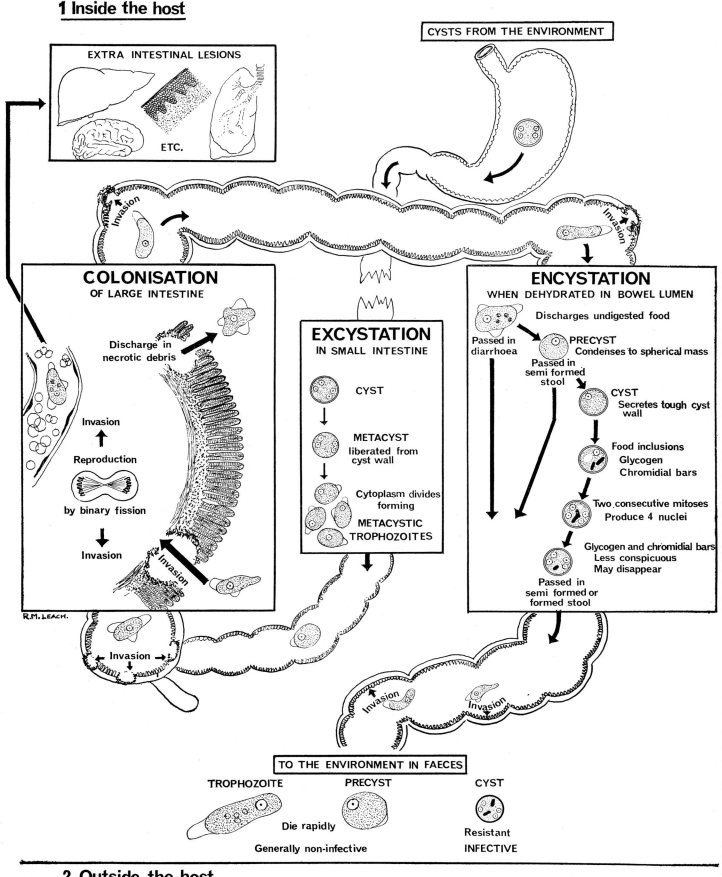

CYSTS FROM THE ENVIRONMENT

EXTRA INTESTINAL LESIONS

ETC.

COLONISATION
OF LARGE INTESTINE

Discharge in necrotic debris

Invasion

Reproduction

by binary fission

Invasion

Invasion

EXCYSTATION
IN SMALL INTESTINE

CYST

METACYST liberated from cyst wall

Cytoplasm divides forming

METACYSTIC TROPHOZOITES

ENCYSTATION
WHEN DEHYDRATED IN BOWEL LUMEN

Discharges undigested food

Passed in diarrhoea

PRECYST Condenses to spherical mass

Passed in semi formed stool

CYST Secretes tough cyst wall

Food inclusions Glycogen Chromidial bars

Two consecutive mitoses Produce 4 nuclei

Glycogen and chromidial bars Less conspicuous May disappear

Passed in semi formed or formed stool

R.M.LEACH.

Invasion

Invasion

Invasion

TO THE ENVIRONMENT IN FAECES

TROPHOZOITE   PRECYST   CYST

Die rapidly   Resistant
Generally non-infective   INFECTIVE

2 Outside the host

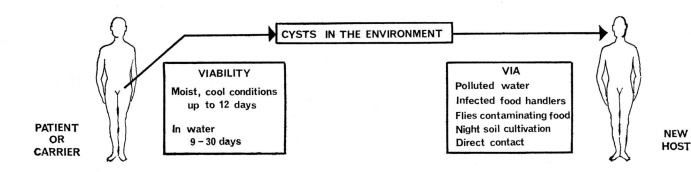

CYSTS IN THE ENVIRONMENT

VIABILITY
Moist, cool conditions up to 12 days
In water 9 – 30 days

VIA
Polluted water
Infected food handlers
Flies contaminating food
Night soil cultivation
Direct contact

PATIENT OR CARRIER

NEW HOST

Entamoeba histolytica

Morphology

PLATE 51

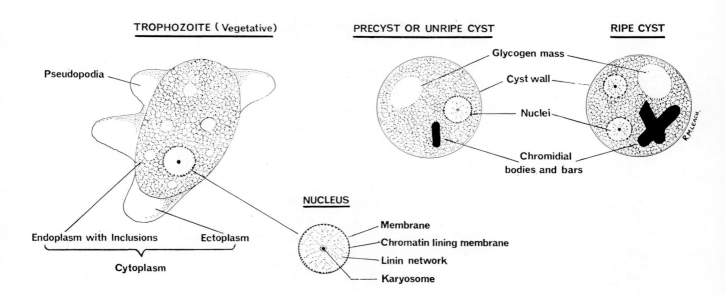

TROPHOZOITE (Vegetative)

Pseudopodia

Endoplasm with Inclusions   Ectoplasm

Cytoplasm

PRECYST OR UNRIPE CYST

RIPE CYST

Glycogen mass

Cyst wall

Nuclei

Chromidial bodies and bars

NUCLEUS

Membrane
Chromatin lining membrane
Linin network
Karyosome

PARTICULAR   Including differentiation from   Entamoeba coli, an intestinal commensal

UNSTAINED PREPARATIONS

E. histolytica   ## E. coli

TROPHOZOITE

E. histolytica	Feature	E. coli
Granular	Cytoplasm	Conspicuously granular
Clear finger-like	Pseudopodia	Blunt
ACTIVE purposeful	Movement	SLUGGISH not purposeful
Generally invisible	Nucleus	Ring refractile granules with eccentric karyosome
RED BLOOD CELLS	Inclusions	Vacuoles, crystals, vegetable cells, bacteria, NO RBC's

15–60 μ   15–50 μ

PRECYST AND UNRIPE CYST

E. histolytica	Feature	E. coli
Granular	Cytoplasm	Granular
May be refractile ring	Nucleus	Visible as refractile ring
Rod-like refractile chromidial bars Glycogen masses	Inclusions	May be slender refractile chromidial bars Glycogen masses

RIPE CYST

E. histolytica	Feature	E. coli
Round	Shape	Round
Refractile	Wall	Conspicuous refractile double outline
Difficult to see (1–4)	Nuclei	1–8 refractile nuclei with eccentric karyosomes
Refractile Chromidial bars often	Inclusions	Only rudimentary slender Chromidial bars

3.5–20 μ   10–33μ

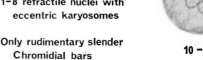

NOTE :

Small race cysts < 10μ. May be commensal (E. hartmanni)

Large race cysts > 10μ. Pathogenic

PLATE 52

Morphology (cont.)

E. histolytica

IODINE PREPARATIONS

E. coli

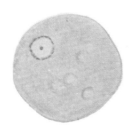

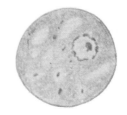

TROPHOZOITE

E. histolytica	Feature	E. coli
Finely granular yellow green	Cytoplasm	Conspicuous granularity
Red cells (yellow)	Inclusions	Bacteria etc. No R.B.C.
Yellow ring with centre yellow dot (Karyosome)	Nucleus	Nuclear membrane with eccentric karyosome easily recognised

PRECYST

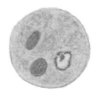

E. histolytica	Feature	E. coli
Brown, diffuse	Glycogen	Brown, compact
As above	Cytoplasm / Nucleus	As above

STAINED BY IRON HAEMATOXYLIN

TROPHOZOITE

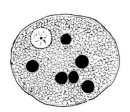

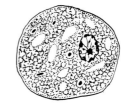

E. histolytica	Feature	E. coli
Purplish brown Faintly granular	Cytoplasm	Greyish blue Coarsely granular
R B C black	Inclusions	Vacuoles black, as are bacteria etc.
Lined with minute black granules	Nucleus Membrane	Thick with plaques of black chromatin
Small black central dot	Karyosome	Eccentric black dot or plaque
Trace only seen	Linin network	More conspicuous may have chromatin plaques

PRECYST

E. histolytica	Feature	E. coli
Round	Shape	Round
As trophozoite	Cytoplasm Nucleus	As trophozoite
Black chromidial bodies or bars	Inclusions	May have slender black chromidial bars
Glycogen (dissolved) replaced by vacuoles		Glycogen (dissolved) replaced by vacuoles

CYST

E. histolytica	Feature	E. coli
Grey- blue	Cytoplasm	Greyish blue, granular
As precyst, less conspicuous or absent	Inclusions	As precyst, less conspicuous or absent In 2 nuclei stage glycogen vacuoles may be dumb bell shaped
Unstained, hyaline	Wall	Unstained, hyaline
As trophozoite 1 - 4	Nuclei	As trophozoite 1 - 8

R.M.Leach.

PLATE 53

Amoebiasis

Pathogenesis

APPARENT SYMBIOSIS

Many harbour E.histolytica with no
   apparent clinical disease

Some authorities say

Small cysts (<10μ) commensal

   E.hartmanni

Large cysts (>10μ) pathogenic

DECREASED
RESISTANCE →

OFFENCE

Cytolytic ferment

Motility   INVASION

Secondary infection

→

DEFENCE

Practically none

Inflammatory reaction

Pathology

1. COLONISATION OF THE LARGE INTESTINE

SITE OF ENTRY

   INITIALLY MINUTE

   THEN IRREGULAR ULCER

SHAPE TYPICALLY FLASK-LIKE

EDGES OVERHANGING

BASE NECROTIC LYSED TISSUE

AMOEBAE INVADING AROUND

DISCHARGE NECROTIC DEBRIS,

   MUCUS AND AMOEBAE

↓

COLONISATION ELSEWHERE
   IN LARGE BOWEL

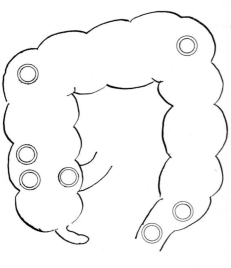

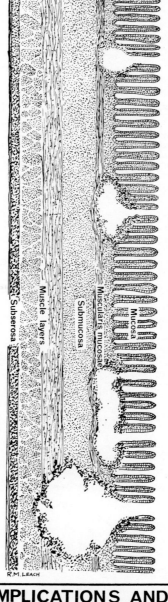

R.M.LEACH

THE PRIMARY ULCER

Invasion of mucosa via crypts

Repair may

   Overtake necrosis — with healing

   Keep pace with necrosis — persistent
      superficial lesions

   Lag behind — extension

EXTENSION IN MUCOSA

Muscularis mucosae relatively
   resistant

Accumulation of amoebae
   superficial to it

Lateral extension of lytic necrosis

FORMATION OF SINUSES

Abscesses may coalesce under
   intact mucosae

Later mucosae may slough with
   widespread ulceration

DEEP EXTENSION

Muscularis mucosae eventually
   pierced (directly or via vessels)

Deep necrosis of sub-mucosa
   even muscle and sub-serosa

2. COMPLICATIONS AND SEQUELAE

PERFORATION
   HAEMORRHAGE (RARE)

SECONDARY INFECTION

AMOEBOMA (RARE)
   (Clinically simulates neoplasm)

INVASION OF BLOOD VESSELS
DIRECT EXTENSION OUTSIDE BOWEL

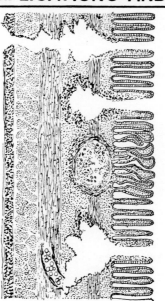

With peritonitis
   haemorrhage

With surrounding inflammatory reaction and fibroblastic
   proliferation

A mass under oedematous mucosa with
   Internal abscesses of necrotic tissue and amoebae
Surrounding granulomatous tissue zone with eosinophils
   lymphocytes and fibroblasts
An outer firm nodular fibrous tissue

3 EXTRA-INTESTINAL LESIONS — PLATE 54

PLATE 54

Pathology of Amoebiasis (cont.)

3. EXTRA-INTESTINAL LESIONS

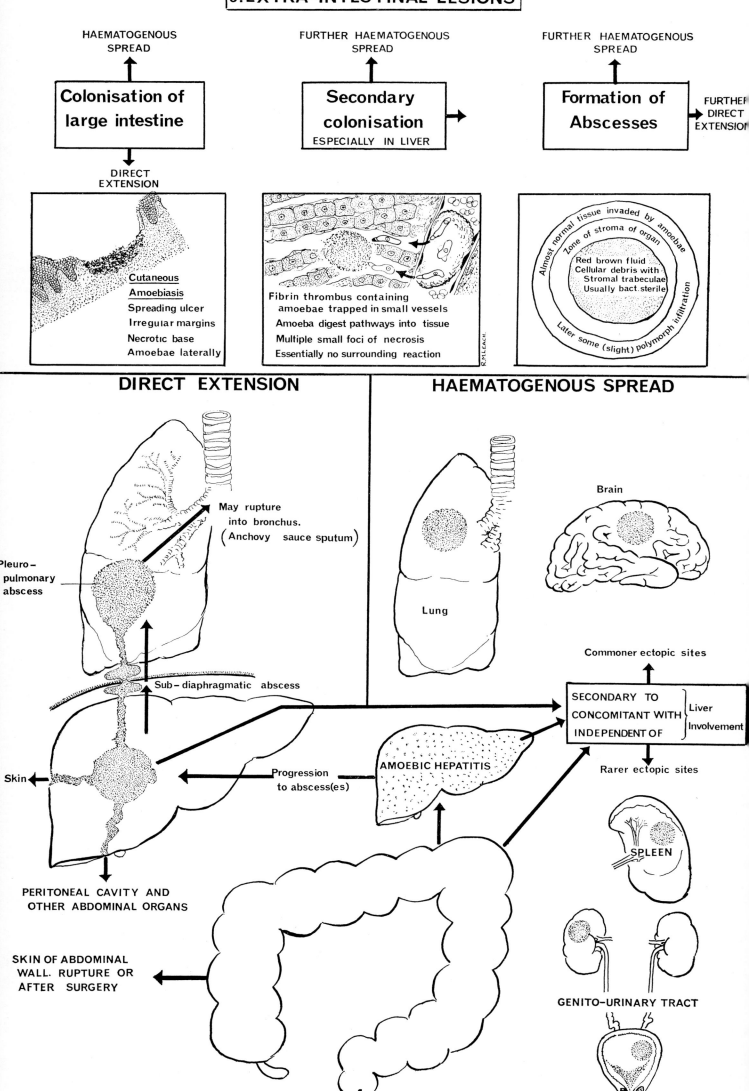

HAEMATOGENOUS SPREAD

Colonisation of large intestine

DIRECT EXTENSION

Cutaneous Amoebiasis
Spreading ulcer
Irregular margins
Necrotic base
Amoebae laterally

FURTHER HAEMATOGENOUS SPREAD

Secondary colonisation
ESPECIALLY IN LIVER

Fibrin thrombus containing amoebae trapped in small vessels
Amoeba digest pathways into tissue
Multiple small foci of necrosis
Essentially no surrounding reaction

FURTHER HAEMATOGENOUS SPREAD

Formation of Abscesses

FURTHER DIRECT EXTENSION

Almost normal tissue invaded by amoebae
Zone of stroma of organ
Red brown fluid
Cellular debris with
Stromal trabeculae
Usually bact. sterile
Later some (slight) polymorph infiltration

R.M.LEACH.

DIRECT EXTENSION

May rupture into bronchus. (Anchovy sauce sputum)

Pleuro-pulmonary abscess

Sub-diaphragmatic abscess

Skin

Progression to abscess(es)

PERITONEAL CAVITY AND OTHER ABDOMINAL ORGANS

SKIN OF ABDOMINAL WALL. RUPTURE OR AFTER SURGERY

HAEMATOGENOUS SPREAD

Brain

Lung

Commoner ectopic sites

SECONDARY TO
CONCOMITANT WITH
INDEPENDENT OF
Liver Involvement

Rarer ectopic sites

AMOEBIC HEPATITIS

SPLEEN

GENITO-URINARY TRACT

PERIANAL SKIN

PLATE 55

Laboratory Diagnosis of Amoebiasis

PRIMARILY DEPENDS ON DEMONSTRATION OF <u>E. histolytica</u> in Stool

> Aspirates, intestinal or other organs
> Biopsy material Pinch biopsy at proctoscopy
> or sigmoidoscopy
> Surgical biopsy elsewhere

INTESTINAL

Stool examination Including differentiation from stool in bacillary dysentery

	AMOEBIASIS	SHIGELLOSIS
NAKED EYE		
Faecal matter	Always present	May be absent. Blood and mucus only
Mucus	Not tenacious	Tenacious
	Not abundant	Abundant in acute stages
MICROSCOPIC		
(1) Bacteria	Numerous	May be scanty
(2) Pus cells	Scanty, well preserved	Very numerous, degenerate
(3) Red blood cells	Often in rouleaux	Scattered

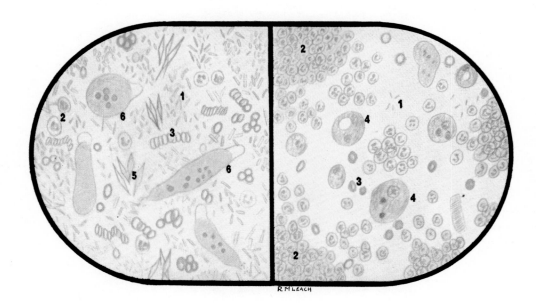

R M LEACH

	AMOEBIASIS	SHIGELLOSIS
(4) Large macrophages	Not a feature	May be numerous, may have ingested red cells (do not mistake for amoebae)
(5) Charcot-Leyden crystals	May be present	Absent
(6) <u>E. histolytica</u>	Present	Absent
CULTURE	Special methods for amoebae (Not employed as a routine)	Isolation of Shigella spp.

Remember

Vegetative <u>Entamoeba histolytica</u> in diarrhoea	ACTIVELY MOTILE PURPOSEFUL MOVEMENT FINGER LIKE CLEAR PSEUDOPODIA INGESTED RED CELLS NO NUCLEUS SEEN
Precyst or cysts in semi-formed or solid stool	NUCLEAR CHARACTERISTICS NUMBER OF NUCLEI (1—4) GLYCOGEN CHROMIDIAL BARS

Serological tests C.F.T. of little value in uncomplicated intestinal amoebiasis

Amoebic hepatitis and abscess

LEUCOCYTOSIS

STOOL EXAMINATION — for <u>E.histolytica</u>

SEROLOGICAL TESTS — C.F.T. using extract of culture of amoebae as antigen : of doubtful value.

ASPIRATED MATERIAL — examination for <u>E.histolytica</u>

BIOPSY MATERIAL — histology

Other extra—intestinal lesions

ALONG SIMILAR LINES

The Non-Pathogenic Intestinal Amoebae

LIFE CYCLE

CYSTS (Vegetative forms of D.fragilis) FROM ENVIRONMENT

EXCYSTATION IN SMALL INTESTINE

ENCYSTATION (except in D.fragilis) if dehydrated

MULTIPLICATION OF VEGETATIVE FORMS IN LARGE INTESTINE

CYSTS (vegetative forms of D.fragilis) TO ENVIRONMENT in formed stools
Vegetative forms found in diarrhoea

MORPHOLOGY

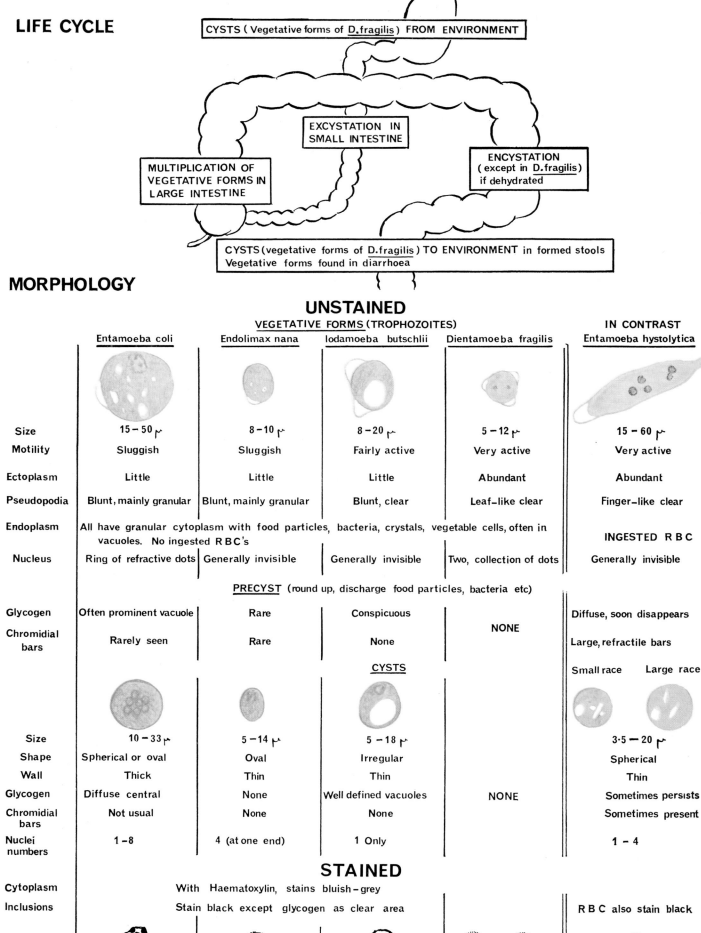

UNSTAINED
VEGETATIVE FORMS (TROPHOZOITES)

	Entamoeba coli	Endolimax nana	Iodamoeba butschlii	Dientamoeba fragilis	IN CONTRAST Entamoeba hystolytica
Size	15 – 50 μ	8 – 10 μ	8 – 20 μ	5 – 12 μ	15 – 60 μ
Motility	Sluggish	Sluggish	Fairly active	Very active	Very active
Ectoplasm	Little	Little	Little	Abundant	Abundant
Pseudopodia	Blunt, mainly granular	Blunt, mainly granular	Blunt, clear	Leaf-like clear	Finger-like clear
Endoplasm	All have granular cytoplasm with food particles, bacteria, crystals, vegetable cells, often in vacuoles. No ingested RBC's				INGESTED R B C
Nucleus	Ring of refractive dots	Generally invisible	Generally invisible	Two, collection of dots	Generally invisible

PRECYST (round up, discharge food particles, bacteria etc)

	Entamoeba coli	Endolimax nana	Iodamoeba butschlii	Dientamoeba fragilis	Entamoeba hystolytica
Glycogen	Often prominent vacuole	Rare	Conspicuous	NONE	Diffuse, soon disappears
Chromidial bars	Rarely seen	Rare	None		Large, refractile bars

CYSTS

	Entamoeba coli	Endolimax nana	Iodamoeba butschlii	Dientamoeba fragilis	Small race / Large race
Size	10 – 33 μ	5 – 14 μ	5 – 18 μ		3·5 – 20 μ
Shape	Spherical or oval	Oval	Irregular		Spherical
Wall	Thick	Thin	Thin		Thin
Glycogen	Diffuse central	None	Well defined vacuoles	NONE	Sometimes persists
Chromidial bars	Not usual	None	None		Sometimes present
Nuclei numbers	1 – 8	4 (at one end)	1 Only		1 – 4

STAINED

	Entamoeba coli	Endolimax nana	Iodamoeba butschlii	Dientamoeba fragilis	Entamoeba hystolytica
Cytoplasm	With Haematoxylin, stains bluish-grey				
Inclusions	Stain black except glycogen as clear area				R B C also stain black

NUCLEAR Characteristics

	Entamoeba coli	Endolimax nana	Iodamoeba butschlii	Dientamoeba fragilis	Entamoeba hystolytica
Membrane	Thick	Thin	Thick	Very delicate	Delicate
Chromatin on membrane	Coarse	None	Sometimes granular	None	Fine granules
Karyosome	Coarse generally eccentric	Large irregular	Large lateral	Central granules	Small central
Linin network	May be chromatin particles	No chromatin	No chromatin	Delicate fibrils	Not often seen

PATHOGENICITY

Entamoeba coli	Endolimax nana	Iodamoeba butschlii	Dientamoeba fragilis	Entamoeba hystolytica
Harmless commensal	Harmless commensal	Usually harmless commensal (One invasive case described)	No evidence of pathogenicity	May be invasive

The Body–Fluid and Tissue Flagellates

PLATE 57

CAUSING LEISHMANIASIS AND TRYPANOSOMIASIS

CLASSIFICATION

Phylum	**PROTOZOA** (Unicellular organisms)
Sub–phylum	Sporozoa Sarcodina **MASTIGOPHORA** (Move by flagella, Asexual reproduction) Ciliophora Uncertain status
Class	**ZOOMASTIGOPHOREA**
Sub-class	**GROUP A** (Live in intestinal tract and genitalia, No vector required) **GROUP B** (Live in blood stream and tissues, Vector (blood sucking invertebrates) required)
Family	**TRYPANOSOMATIDAE** (Single flagellum)

POSTERIOR — Undulating membrane, Axoneme, Kinetoplast, Nucleus, Volutin granules, Flagellum — ANTERIOR

MORPHOLOGICAL STAGES OF TRYPANOSOMATIDAE; GENERA AND SPECIES AFFECTING MAN

AMASTIGOTE (LEISHMANIAL)	PROMASTIGOTE (LEPTOMONAD)	EPIMASTIGOTE (CRITHIDIAL)	TRYPOMASTIGOTE (TRYPANOSOMAL)
Intracellular in macrophages of man	In midgut then proboscis of sandfly. TRANSFER STAGE TO MAN (Also in culture)		
LEISHMANIA DONOVANI _LEISHMANIA TROPICA_ _LEISHMANIA BRAZILIENSIS_			
		In salivary glands of Tsetse fly.	In midgut, salivary glands and proboscis of tsetse fly. TRANSFER STAGE TO MAN. In blood stream, lymph nodes and later C.N.S. of man.
			TRYPANOSOMA RHODESIENSE _TRYPANOSOMA GAMBIENSE_
Intracellular in macrophages and tissue cells of man.	Transitional stage only	In midgut of bug	In midgut of bug. In faeces of bug. TRANSFER STAGE TO MAN. In blood and tissue spaces of man.
		TRYPANOSOMA CRUZI	

R.M.LEACH.

Leishmaniasis

PLATE 58

Species	L.DONOVANI	L.TROPICA	L.BRAZILIENSIS
Disease	VISCERAL (KALA AZAR)	CUTANEOUS (ORIENTAL SORE)	MUCO-CUTANEOUS (ESPUNDIA)

Life cycle and morphology of leishmania (SIMILAR IN ALL THREE SPECIES)

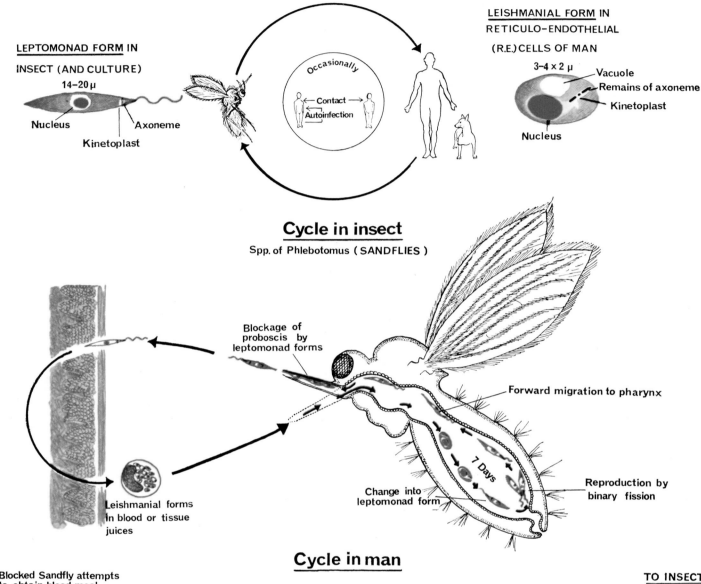

LEPTOMONAD FORM IN INSECT (AND CULTURE)
14–20 μ
Nucleus
Axoneme
Kinetoplast

Occasionally
Contact
Autoinfection

LEISHMANIAL FORM IN RETICULO-ENDOTHELIAL (R.E.) CELLS OF MAN
3–4 × 2 μ
Vacuole
Remains of axoneme
Kinetoplast
Nucleus

Cycle in insect
Spp. of Phlebotomus (SANDFLIES)

Blockage of proboscis by leptomonad forms

Forward migration to pharynx

7 Days

Change into leptomonad form

Reproduction by binary fission

Leishmanial forms in blood or tissue juices

Cycle in man

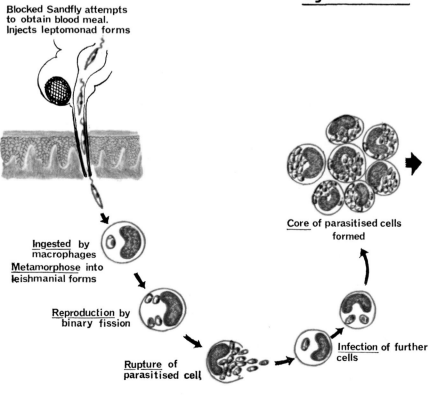

Blocked Sandfly attempts to obtain blood meal. Injects leptomonad forms

Ingested by macrophages
Metamorphose into leishmanial forms

Reproduction by binary fission

Rupture of parasitised cell

Infection of further cells

Core of parasitised cells formed

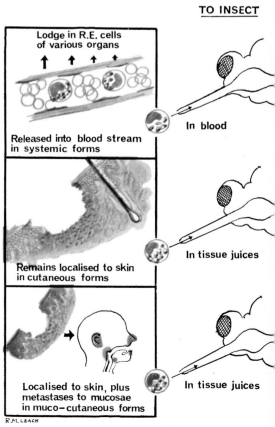

TO INSECT

Lodge in R.E. cells of various organs

Released into blood stream in systemic forms

In blood

Remains localised to skin in cutaneous forms

In tissue juices

Localised to skin, plus metastases to mucosae in muco-cutaneous forms

In tissue juices

R.M. LEACH

PLATE 59

Visceral Leishmaniasis (Kala Azar)

CAUSED BY LEISHMANIA DONOVANI

PATHOGENESIS AND PATHOLOGY

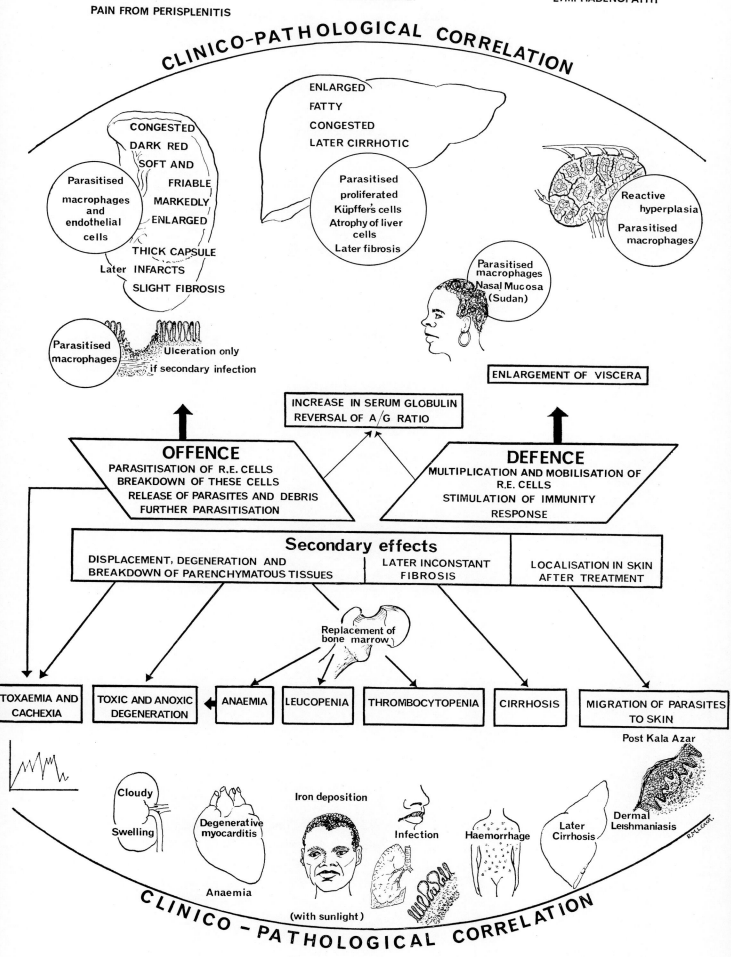

SPLENOMEGALY   HEPATOMEGALY   LYMPHADENOPATHY

PAIN FROM PERISPLENITIS

CLINICO-PATHOLOGICAL CORRELATION

CONGESTED
DARK RED
SOFT AND
FRIABLE
MARKEDLY
ENLARGED
THICK CAPSULE
Later INFARCTS
SLIGHT FIBROSIS

Parasitised macrophages and endothelial cells

ENLARGED
FATTY
CONGESTED
LATER CIRRHOTIC

Parasitised proliferated Küpffer's cells Atrophy of liver cells Later fibrosis

Reactive hyperplasia Parasitised macrophages

Parasitised macrophages Nasal Mucosa (Sudan)

Parasitised macrophages — Ulceration only if secondary infection

ENLARGEMENT OF VISCERA

INCREASE IN SERUM GLOBULIN
REVERSAL OF A/G RATIO

OFFENCE
PARASITISATION OF R.E. CELLS
BREAKDOWN OF THESE CELLS
RELEASE OF PARASITES AND DEBRIS
FURTHER PARASITISATION

DEFENCE
MULTIPLICATION AND MOBILISATION OF R.E. CELLS
STIMULATION OF IMMUNITY
RESPONSE

Secondary effects

DISPLACEMENT, DEGENERATION AND BREAKDOWN OF PARENCHYMATOUS TISSUES | LATER INCONSTANT FIBROSIS | LOCALISATION IN SKIN AFTER TREATMENT

Replacement of bone marrow

TOXAEMIA AND CACHEXIA | TOXIC AND ANOXIC DEGENERATION | ANAEMIA | LEUCOPENIA | THROMBOCYTOPENIA | CIRRHOSIS | MIGRATION OF PARASITES TO SKIN

Post Kala Azar

Cloudy Swelling

Degenerative myocarditis

Iron deposition

Infection

Haemorrhage

Later Cirrhosis

Dermal Leishmaniasis

Anaemia

(with sunlight)

CLINICO-PATHOLOGICAL CORRELATION

Fever	Albuminuria	Pallor	Darkening of skin	Stomatitis	Purpura		Later
Weakness		Cardiac dilatation	forehead, temples	Cancrum oris	Epistaxis	Jaundice	Macular, papular,
Loss of weight		Tachycardia	around mouth	Cough etc.	Melaena	Ascites	or nodular
E.S.R. raised		Low B.P.	(Kala azar =	Diarrhoea			rashes
		Haemic murmurs	Black fever)				
		Ankle oedema					

Cutaneous Leishmaniasis

PLATE 60

(Oriental sore, Chiclero's disease, Uta etc.)

Caused by Leishmania tropica

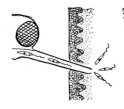 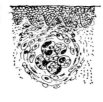 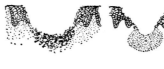 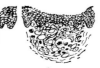 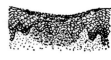

Blocked sandfly injects leptomonad forms | Core of cells parasitised by L.D. bodies formed — Remains localised to skin | Acanthosis cellular infiltration | Pressure necrosis and ulceration — Ulcer with sharp cut edges and surrounding induration | Secondary infection | Granulation | Healing (2–12 months) with depressed pigmented scar

Muco-cutaneous Leishmaniasis (Espundia)
Caused by Leishmania braziliensis

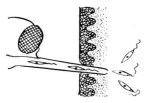 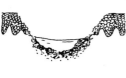 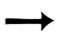 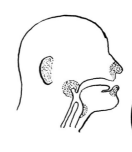

Blocked sandfly injects leptomonad forms | Cutaneous manifestations like oriental sore but often weeping ulcers | Spread to mucosae of Mouth·Nose, Larynx, Pharynx, Ear. | Parasitised cells Inflammatory infiltration Necrosis Later reactive fibrosis

SECONDARY EFFECTS IN LOOSE MUCOSAL TISSUES

| Oedema and capillary involvement Interference with local blood supply Necrosis — Extensive destruction | Secondary infection Deep erosion locally Spread of infection to lungs or elsewhere | Healing with fibrosis |

Leading to

Extensive disfiguring lesions | General constitutional upset (fever, pain, anaemia.) | Broncho–pneumonia and septicaemia

DIAGNOSIS OF LEISHMANIASIS

Visceral

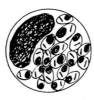

1. DEMONSTRATION OF PARASITE by Stained film / Culture (N.N.N.) / Animal inoculation (Hamsters) — in Blood, Bone Marrow, Lymph node juice, Nasal scrapings (Sudan), Spleen puncture } not free from danger, Liver puncture

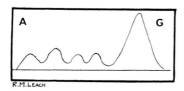

2. SEROLOGICAL TESTS — Specific: C.F.T. (Antigen, leishmania cultures) — Non-specific: Depending on reversal A G ratio, Formal gel (Napier), Aldehyde (Chopra), Euglobulin precipitation (Sia), Electrophoresis

R.M.LEACH.

Cutaneous and Muco-cutaneous

1. Demonstration of parasite by Stained film / Culture / Animal inoculation — in Serum from indurated edge of ulcer, Biopsy of margin of ulcer, Mucosal scraping in mucocutaneous type

2. Intradermal test (Montenegro), Antigen culture of appropriate leishmania

3. Serological tests in muco-cutaneous type

Trypanosomiasis

PLATE 61

African type : Sleeping sickness

CAUSED BY either Trypanosoma gambiense (Chronic sleeping sickness)   Similar morphology
Trypanosoma rhodesiense (Acute sleeping sickness)   and life cycle

MORPHOLOGY

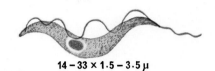

14 – 33 × 1.5 – 3.5 μ

VARIATIONS

Short stumpy aflagellate forms in blood

Involution (round or pear shaped) forms in C.S.F.

Crithidial form at one stage in vector

LIFE CYCLE : GENERAL

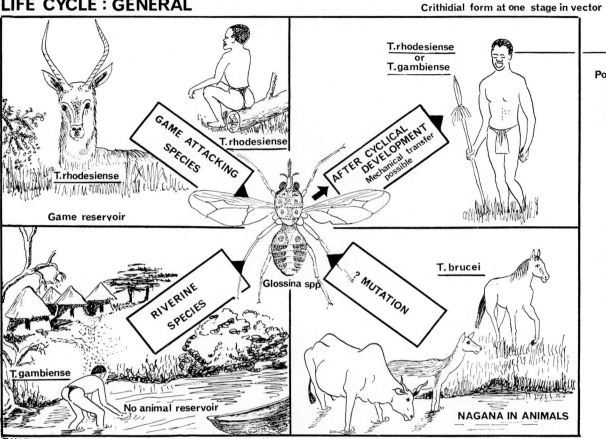

GAME ATTACKING SPECIES

T.rhodesiense

Game reservoir

T.rhodesiense

AFTER CYCLICAL DEVELOPMENT
Mechanical transfer possible

T.rhodesiense or T.gambiense

Possibly congenital or by coitus

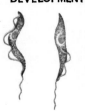

RIVERINE SPECIES

Glossina spp

? MUTATION

T. brucei

T.gambiense

No animal reservoir

NAGANA IN ANIMALS

R.M.LEACH.

LIFE CYCLE : IN INSECT

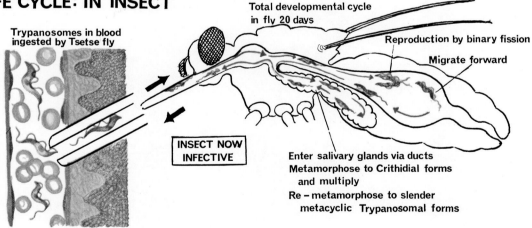

Total developmental cycle in fly **20 days**

Reproduction by binary fission

Migrate forward

Trypanosomes in blood ingested by Tsetse fly

INSECT NOW INFECTIVE

Enter salivary glands via ducts
Metamorphose to Crithidial forms and multiply
Re – metamorphose to slender metacyclic Trypanosomal forms

ANTERIOR STATION DEVELOPMENT

LIFE CYCLE : IN MAN

REPRODUCTION BY BINARY FISSION AS TRYPANOSOMAL FORMS

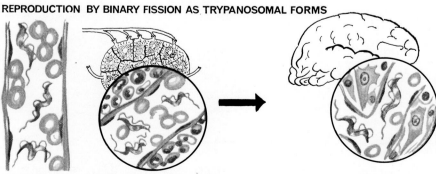

Metacyclic Trypanosomes injected by Tse tse fly

Multiply at site of injection

Invade blood stream

and tissue spaces of various organs particularly lymph nodes initially

But do NOT enter actual cells

Then C.N.S.

PRIMARY STAGE   **SECONDARY STAGE**   **THIRD STAGE**

PLATE 62

African Trypanosomiasis (Sleeping Sickness) continued
Pathogenesis and Pathology

PRIMARY STAGE   **SECONDARY STAGE**   **THIRD STAGE**

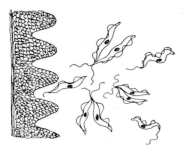

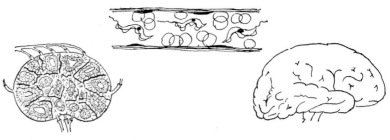

Multiplication at site of injection
Surrounding inflammatory reaction

Parasitaemia and Toxaemia
Invasion of tissue spaces (NOT cells) of various organs.
Predominantly
Lymph nodes   C.N.S.
Damage to endothelial cells of blood vessels, surrounding
(perivascular) granulomatous reactions and haemorrhages.

| LOCAL INFLAMMATORY LESION Usually only seen in Europeans |
| TOXIC DEGENERATION AND PRESSURE ATROPHY OF TISSUE CELLS |

Chronic Sleeping Sickness
(Due to T. gambiense)

DIFFER ONLY IN DEGREE

Acute Sleeping Sickness
(Due to T. rhodesiense)

CLINICO–PATHOLOGICAL CORRELATION

STAGE — PRIMARY

CLINICO–PATHOLOGICAL CORRELATION

Firm, tender painful red nodule 1–3 weeks.

TRYPANOSOMAL CHANCRE   TRYPANOSOMAL CHANCRE

As in chronic

SECONDARY
PREDOMINANTLY BLOOD AND LYMPH NODE INVOLVEMENT

FEVER
Low.
Irregular.
Recurrent.
General toxic
    symptoms.
Backache.
Headache.
Tachycardia.
Irregular skin
    rashes.
Transient oedema
    face

LYMPHADENOPATHY
Typically
    post–cervical.
Later anaemia
    monocytosis.
Slight enlargement
    liver, spleen.

Enlarged Soft Red
Later Regress Fibrotic
Congestion Sinus catarrh Perivascular cuffing

Congested Slightly enlarged
Toxic depression Bone marrow

Similar lesions not so pronounced

Toxic depression Bone marrow

Slightly enlarged

FEVER
High
Persistent

SEVERE TOXIC SYMPTOMS
Headache
Vomiting
Shivering
Oedema face
Serous effusion
Bone pain
Lymphadenopathy

ANAEMIA
PURPURA

often DEATH

at this stage

THIRD – C.N.S. INVOLVEMENT

PROGRESSIVE INVOLVEMENT of the **CENTRAL NERVOUS SYSTEM**

Generalised leptomeningitis.
Dura thickened and adherent.
Oedema with flat convolutions.
    and dilated ventricles,
Haemorrhage with softening.
C.S.F. turbid, increase cells and protein,
    containing trypanosomes.

General symptoms
of an organic
    encephalitis.
Focal signs
    uncommon.

Perivascular cuffing
with round and plasma
cells, macrophages and
endothelial cells.
Neuroglial proliferation.
Pressure atrophy
    neurones.

Death before C.N.S. involvement
or
similar changes
but more acute

May have
early onset of
encephalitis
with rapid
development of
COMA.

Note on epidemiology

Vectors of T. gambiense are RIVERINE species, hence
disease often epidemic.
G. palpalis
G. tachinoides

Vectors of T. rhodesiense are GAME–ATTACKING species, disease
more often sporadic.
G. morsitans
G. pallidipes
G. swynnertoni

PLATE 63

Trypanosomiasis
South American Type: Chaga's Disease
Caused by Trypanosoma cruzi

Life cycle: General

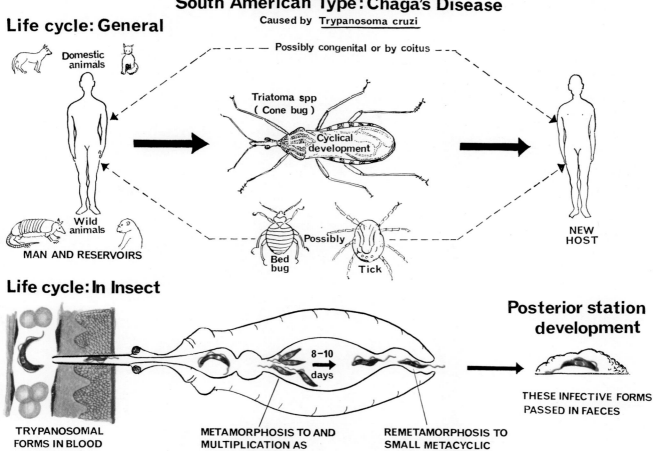

Domestic animals

Possibly congenital or by coitus

Triatoma spp (Cone bug)

Cyclical development

Wild animals

MAN AND RESERVOIRS

Possibly

Bed bug

Tick

NEW HOST

Life cycle: In Insect

Posterior station development

8-10 days

THESE INFECTIVE FORMS PASSED IN FAECES

TRYPANOSOMAL FORMS IN BLOOD INGESTED BY BUG

METAMORPHOSIS TO AND MULTIPLICATION AS CRITHIDIAL FORMS

REMETAMORPHOSIS TO SMALL METACYCLIC TRYPANOSOMAL FORMS

Life cycle: In Man

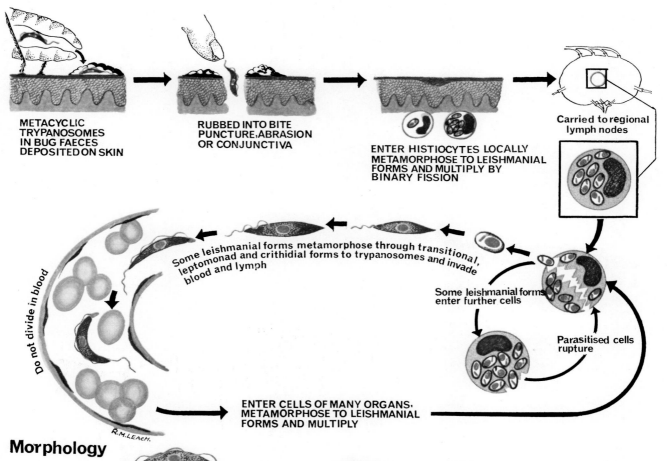

METACYCLIC TRYPANOSOMES IN BUG FAECES DEPOSITED ON SKIN

RUBBED INTO BITE PUNCTURE, ABRASION OR CONJUNCTIVA

ENTER HISTIOCYTES LOCALLY METAMORPHOSE TO LEISHMANIAL FORMS AND MULTIPLY BY BINARY FISSION

Carried to regional lymph nodes

Some leishmanial forms metamorphose through transitional, leptomonad and crithidial forms to trypanosomes and invade blood and lymph

Some leishmanial forms enter further cells

Parasitised cells rupture

Do not divide in blood

ENTER CELLS OF MANY ORGANS, METAMORPHOSE TO LEISHMANIAL FORMS AND MULTIPLY

R.M.LEACH.

Morphology

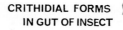

Axoneme

Small parabasal body

Large blepharoplast

TRYPANOSOMAL FORMS IN BLOOD OF MAN AND GUT OF INSECT
Resemble African trypanosomes except Characteristic C shape. Conspicuous kinetoplast. Long and short forms may occur.

LEISHMANIAL FORMS IN CELLS OF MAN
Indistinguishable (except for site) from Leishman-donovan bodies of leishmaniasis.

CRITHIDIAL FORMS IN GUT OF INSECT
and transitional stage in man.

LEPTOMONAD FORMS
transitional only in man

PLATE 6

South American Trypanosomiasis (Chaga's disease) continued

Pathogenesis and Pathology

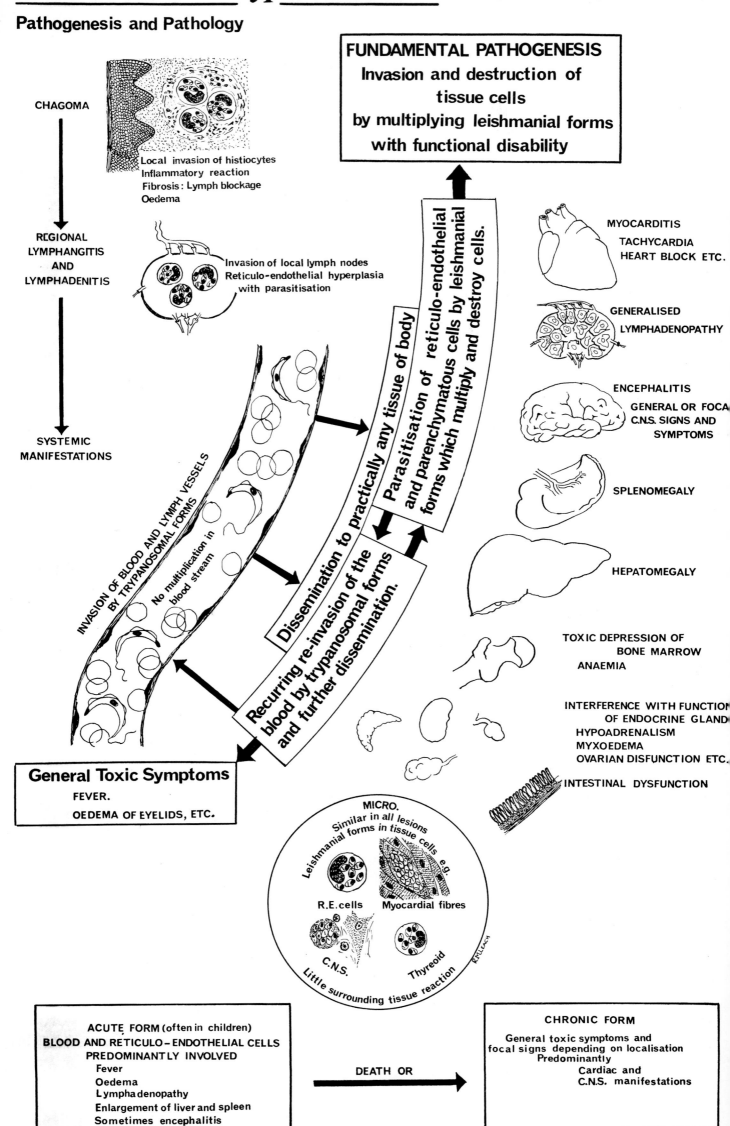

CHAGOMA

Local invasion of histiocytes
Inflammatory reaction
Fibrosis: Lymph blockage
Oedema

REGIONAL
LYMPHANGITIS
AND
LYMPHADENITIS

Invasion of local lymph nodes
Reticulo-endothelial hyperplasia
with parasitisation

SYSTEMIC
MANIFESTATIONS

INVASION OF BLOOD AND LYMPH VESSELS
BY TRYPANOSOMAL FORMS

No multiplication in blood stream

Dissemination to practically any tissue of body

Recurring re-invasion of the blood by trypanosomal forms and further dissemination.

Parasitisation of reticulo-endothelial and parenchymatous cells by leishmanial forms which multiply and destroy cells.

FUNDAMENTAL PATHOGENESIS
Invasion and destruction of tissue cells
by multiplying leishmanial forms
with functional disability

MYOCARDITIS
TACHYCARDIA
HEART BLOCK ETC.

GENERALISED
LYMPHADENOPATHY

ENCEPHALITIS
GENERAL OR FOCAL
C.N.S. SIGNS AND
SYMPTOMS

SPLENOMEGALY

HEPATOMEGALY

TOXIC DEPRESSION OF
BONE MARROW
ANAEMIA

INTERFERENCE WITH FUNCTION
OF ENDOCRINE GLANDS
HYPOADRENALISM
MYXOEDEMA
OVARIAN DISFUNCTION ETC.

INTESTINAL DYSFUNCTION

General Toxic Symptoms
FEVER.
OEDEMA OF EYELIDS, ETC.

MICRO.
Similar in all lesions
Leishmanial forms in tissue cells e.g.
R.E. cells
Myocardial fibres
C.N.S.
Thyreoid
Little surrounding tissue reaction

ACUTE FORM (often in children)
BLOOD AND RETICULO-ENDOTHELIAL CELLS
PREDOMINANTLY INVOLVED
Fever
Oedema
Lymphadenopathy
Enlargement of liver and spleen
Sometimes encephalitis

DEATH OR

CHRONIC FORM
General toxic symptoms and
focal signs depending on localisation
Predominantly
Cardiac and
C.N.S. manifestations

PLATE 65

Trypanosomiasis

LABORATORY DIAGNOSIS

African Type

(SLEEPING SICKNESS)

1 DEMONSTRATION OF THE PARASITE

Fresh preparations

BY
- Stained films —
  - Thick
  - Thin
  - Concentration methods
- Animal inoculation. (T. rhodesiense)
- Culture (possible but difficult)

FROM
- Blood
- Bone marrow
- Lymph node juice
- Cerebro — spinal fluid

successively

2 SEROLOGICAL METHODS

A complement fixation test for T. gambiense now available

Formol gel test (as for Leishmaniasis) may be positive

Note: Paul – Bunnell test (for heterophile antibodies) may be positive

South American Type

(CHAGA'S DISEASE)

1 DEMONSTRATION OF THE PARASITE

BY
- Fresh preparations
- Stained films
- Animal inoculation
- Culture
- Xenodiagnosis

- Histological techniques

FROM
- Blood (Trypanosomal forms)
- Lymph node juice (Leishmanial forms)
- Blood
- Lymph node juice (Trypanosomal forms)
- Blood (Clean bred triatomid bugs fed on patient or his blood develop Trypanosomes in gut)
- Biopsy material
- Post – mortem material

2 SEROLOGICAL METHODS

Specific Complement Fixation Test available

Recapitulation

PLATE 66

THE ESSENTIAL DIFFERENCES BETWEEN :

	AFRICAN TRYPANOSOMIASIS (Sleeping sickness)	SOUTH AMERICAN TRYPANOSOMIASIS (Chaga's disease)	VISCERAL LEISHMANIASIS (Kala Azar)
CAUSED BY	Trypanosoma gambiense or Trypanosoma rhodesiense	Trypanosoma cruzi	Leishmania donovani
VECTOR	Glossina spp. (tsetse flies)	Triatomida spp. (cone-nosed bugs)	Phlebotomus spp. (sandflies)
CYCLE IN VECTOR	Anterior station development	Posterior station development	Anterior station development
Stage ingested	Trypanosomal	Trypanosomal	Leishmanial
Then	Multiply and move forward Enter salivary glands via duct Metamorphoso to Crithidia Multiply Metamorphose to metacyclic Trypanosomes INFECTIVE : INJECTED IN SALIVA	Metamorphose to Crithidia Multiply Move backward Metamorphose to metacyclic Trypanosomes INFECTIVE : PASSED IN BUG FAECES	Metamorphose to Leptomonad Multiply Move forward Block proboscis INFECTIVE: INJECTED FROM PROBOSCIS
CYCLE IN MAN			
Form injected	Metacyclic Trypanosome	Metacyclic Trypanosome	Leptomonad
Metamorphosis	NONE – remain as Trypanosomes	Enter histiocytes locally and become Leishmanial	Enter histiocytes locally and become Leishmanial
Multiplication (all by binary fision)	as TRYPANOSOMES in BLOOD and tissue spaces	As Leishmanial forms in cells	As Leishmanial forms in macrophage cells
Then	Remain in blood stream as Trypanosomes	Carried to regional nodes : some Leishmanial forms infect further histiocytes : some metamorphose through transitional Leptomonad and Crithidial forms to gain blood as Trypanosomes. Do not multiply as such but disseminated, enter further tissue cells, metamorphose to Leishmanial forms and multiply	Further dissemination as Leishmanial forms ONLY
PATHOGENESIS	Circulating, multiplying Trypanosomes cause Parasitaemia and Toxaemia, damaging tissues	Parasitisation and destruction of all types of tissue cells Circulating Trypanosomes produce toxaemia	Parasitisation and destruction of R.E. cells
PATHOLOGICAL EFFECTS	Mainly general toxaemia lymphadenopathy C.N.S involvement	General toxaemia Local functional disability of whichever tissues invaded, especially lymph nodes, heart, C N S	General toxaemia from breakdown of R.E. cells Proliferation of R.E. cells (mainly spleen, liver, bone marrow, lymph nodes) No C.N.S involvement
CLINICO - PATHOLOGICAL CORRELATION	Acute (T. rhodesiense) Fever and severe toxaemia Chronic (T. gambiense) Fever Lymphadenopathy Encephalitis	Fever Enlarged nodes, spleen and liver Protean manifestations depending on localisation in tissues especially Cardiac C.N.S syndromes	Fever Anaemia Enlarged liver and spleen

PLATE 67

Distinction between human and animal trypanosomes (AFTER HOARE)

In epidemiological surveys of infection rates of trypanosomes in vectors (e.g. Glossina spp.), domestic animals or game reservoirs (e.g. Antelopes), certain animal or reptilian trypanosomes may be found and require differentiation from human trypanosomes

GROUPS, SUB GROUPS AND SPECIES

MORPHOLOGICAL VARIATIONS IN	Brucei – Evansi	Vivax	Congolense	Lewisi
Size	18–42 µ	12–20 or 20–26 µ	9–18 or 12–24 µ	Varies 20–90 µ
Shape	POLYMORPHIC (various forms encountered)	MONOMORPHIC (all one form)	MONOMORPHIC or POLYMORPHIC	MONOMORPHIC for spp.
Posterior end	BLUNT (except in slender forms)	BLUNT	BLUNT	POINTED
Kinetoplast	SMALL (none in T. equinum) : typically SUBTERMINAL	LARGE, generally TERMINAL	MEDIUM, typically MARGINAL	VERY LARGE, TERMINAL or SUBTERMINAL
Undulating membrane	CONSPICUOUS	INCONSPICUOUS	CONSPICUOUS or INCONSPICUOUS	INCONSPICUOUS (except in T.grayi and T.theileri)
Free flagellum	PRESENT (except in stumpy forms)	PRESENT	ABSENT or VERY SHORT	PRESENT
Nucleus	CENTRAL (except in post-nucleate forms)	CENTRAL	CENTRAL	CENTRAL (anterior in T.lewisi)
FORMS		SPP.	SPP. and FORMS	SPP.

Brucei

Always POLYMORPHIC
slender and stumpy forms plus others

T. gambiense. In man and Tse tse flies

T. rhodesiense. In man, Tsetse flies and game

T. brucei. In cattle, Tse tse flies and game

slender 29–42 µ
intermediate average 23 µ

Evansi

Polymorphism INCONSTANT
always slender forms, stumpy rare

T. evansi. In domestic animals

T. equinum. } In horses
T. equiperdum. }

stumpy average 18 µ
post-nucleate

T. vivax. } In domestic animals, Tse tse
T. uniforme. } flies and game

T.uniforme 12–20 µ
T.vivax 20–26 µ

T.congolense. In domestic animals and game
T.simiae. In pigs, sometimes in Tse tse flies

T.congolense 9–24 µ
Monomorphic
Polymorphic
slender
short
stout
T.simiae 12–24 µ

T.cruzi. In man, animals and bugs
T.grayi. In crocodiles and Tse tse flies
T.lewisi. In rats
T.theileri. In cattle and game

T.cruzi 20 µ
T.lewisi 25 µ
T.grayi 90 µ
T.theileri 70 µ

PLATE 68

The Intestinal Flagellates

Giardia lamblia

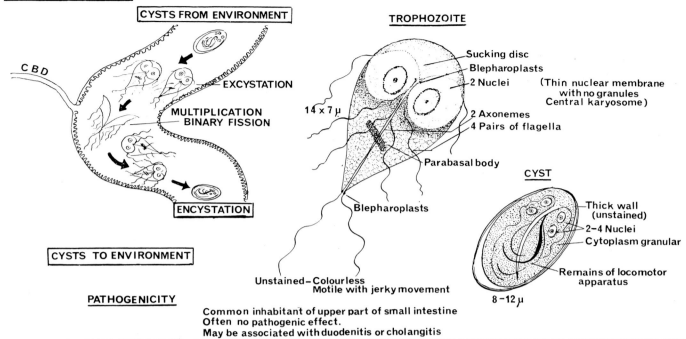

CYSTS FROM ENVIRONMENT

C B D

EXCYSTATION

MULTIPLICATION
BINARY FISSION

ENCYSTATION

CYSTS TO ENVIRONMENT

TROPHOZOITE

Sucking disc
Blepharoplasts
2 Nuclei (Thin nuclear membrane
with no granules
Central karyosome)
2 Axonemes
4 Pairs of flagella
14 x 7 μ
Parabasal body

Blepharoplasts

Unstained–Colourless
Motile with jerky movement

CYST

Thick wall
(unstained)
2–4 Nuclei
Cytoplasm granular
Remains of locomotor
apparatus
8 – 12 μ

PATHOGENICITY

Common inhabitant of upper part of small intestine
Often no pathogenic effect.
May be associated with duodenitis or cholangitis

Chilomastix mesnili

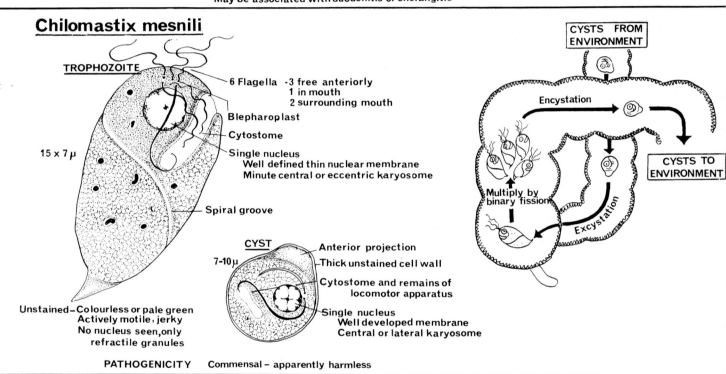

TROPHOZOITE

6 Flagella - 3 free anteriorly
1 in mouth
2 surrounding mouth
Blepharoplast
Cytostome
Single nucleus
Well defined thin nuclear membrane
Minute central or eccentric karyosome

15 x 7 μ

Spiral groove

CYST
7-10 μ

Anterior projection
Thick unstained cell wall
Cytostome and remains of
locomotor apparatus
Single nucleus
Well developed membrane
Central or lateral karyosome

CYSTS FROM
ENVIRONMENT

Encystation

Multiply by
binary fission

Excystation

CYSTS TO
ENVIRONMENT

Unstained–Colourless or pale green
Actively motile, jerky
No nucleus seen, only
refractile granules

PATHOGENICITY   Commensal - apparently harmless

Trichomonas spp.

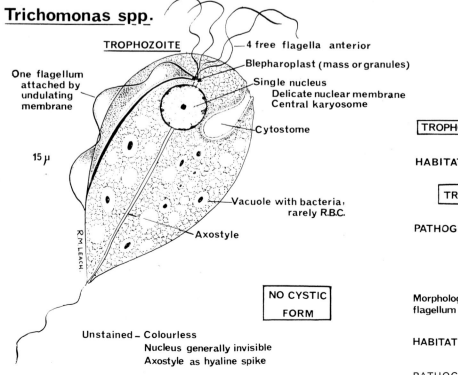

TROPHOZOITE

4 free flagella anterior
Blepharoplast (mass or granules)
Single nucleus
Delicate nuclear membrane
Central karyosome
Cytostome

One flagellum
attached by
undulating
membrane

15 μ

Vacuole with bacteria,
rarely R.B.C.

Axostyle

R.M.LEACH

NO CYSTIC
FORM

Unstained – Colourless
Nucleus generally invisible
Axostyle as hyaline spike

T. hominis (As illustrated)

TROPHOZOITES FROM DAMP ENVIRONMENT

HABITAT   Small and large intestine

TROPHOZOITES TO ENVIRONMENT

PATHOGENICITY Found in diarrhoea but no
proof that it is pathogenic

T. vaginalis

Morphologically as T. hominis but no free posterior
flagellum beyond undulating membrane
Marked parabasal body

HABITAT   Urethra in ♂
Vagina in ♀

PATHOGENICITY   Possible cause of non-specific
urethritis and vaginitis

Balantidium coli
(Causing balantidiasis)

PLATE 69

Classification

Class

PROTOZOA
|
Ciliata
Move by cilia

Generally have mouth (cytosome)

Oesophagus and anal opening
|
Balantidium

Genus

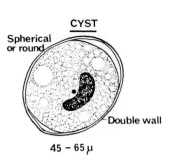

CYST

Spherical or round

Double wall

45 – 65 μ

Ovoid

Coarse cilia

Contractile vacuoles

Horseshoe or kidney shaped macronucleus

Reproduce by binary fission

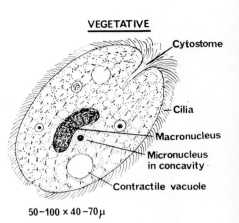

VEGETATIVE

Cytostome

Cilia

Macronucleus

Micronucleus in concavity

Contractile vacuole

50−100 × 40−70 μ

Life cycle

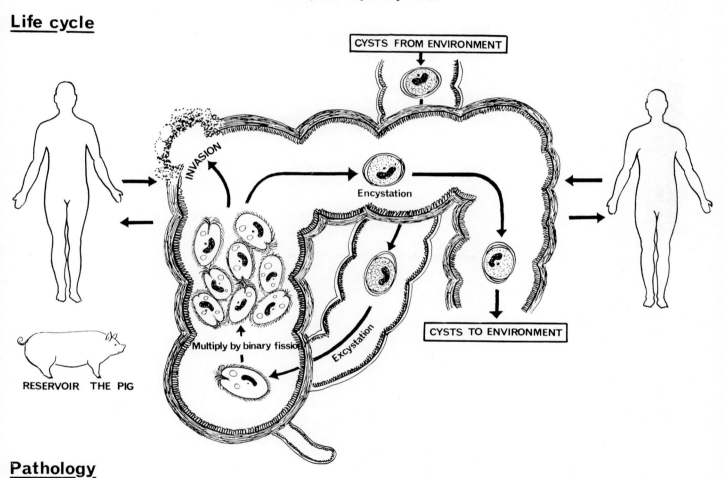

CYSTS FROM ENVIRONMENT

INVASION

Encystation

Excystation

Multiply by binary fission

CYSTS TO ENVIRONMENT

RESERVOIR THE PIG

Pathology

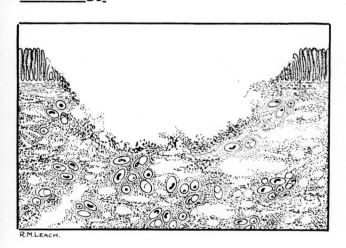

R.M.LEACH.

INVADE like E.histolytica by { MOTILITY / CYTOLYTIC FERMENT

ULCERS wider−mouthed than in amoebic dysentery

SECONDARY INFECTION frequent so cellular infiltration around

LOCALISED to intestine

NO extra-intestinal spread

COMPLICATIONS -perforation

Laboratory diagnosis

Trophozoites in diarrhoea

Cysts in semi-formed and formed stools

PLATE 70

Protozoa of Uncertain Status
Toxoplasma gondii

RESEMBLES <u>PLASMODIUM</u> but
1. Divides by binary fission rather than by schizogony
2. Is non-specific with reference to host and tissue
3. No evidence of an arthropod acting as biological vector
4. Lacks a sexual stage

Morphology

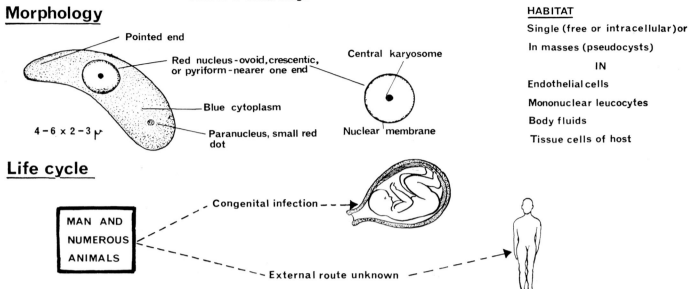

- Pointed end
- Red nucleus - ovoid, crescentic, or pyriform - nearer one end
- Central karyosome
- Blue cytoplasm
- Paranucleus, small red dot
- Nuclear membrane
- 4-6 x 2-3 μ

HABITAT
Single (free or intracellular) or
In masses (pseudocysts)
IN
Endothelial cells
Mononuclear leucocytes
Body fluids
Tissue cells of host

Life cycle

MAN AND NUMEROUS ANIMALS
- Congenital infection
- External route unknown

Pathology
Characteristic association with cells of R.E.system and endothelium of vascular system

CONGENITAL INFECTION
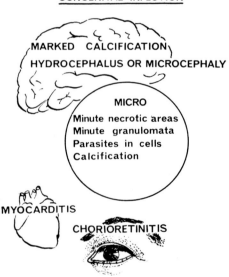
MARKED CALCIFICATION
HYDROCEPHALUS OR MICROCEPHALY
MICRO
Minute necrotic areas
Minute granulomata
Parasites in cells
Calcification
MYOCARDITIS
CHORIORETINITIS

OTHER ROUTES OF INFECTION
INAPPARENT EFFECT
Woman may have affected child though herself show no signs of disease

FEBRILE SYNDROME
Acute fever
Atypical pneumonia
CONGESTED
MICRO
Atypical pneumonia
Parasitised mononuclears in bronchi
Serous effusions

ACUTE ENCEPHALITIS
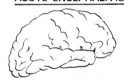
CHORIORETINITIS

LYMPHADENOPATHY
ENLARGED
MICRO
Reactive Hyperplasia
Conspicuous collections of histiocytes

Laboratory diagnosis

DEMONSTRATION OF PARASITE
FROM { Post mortem / Ventricular aspirate / Biopsy liver and spleen } BY } Animal inoculation

SEROLOGICAL: DEMONSTRATION OF SPECIFIC ANTIBODIES
BY - Complement fixation / Neutralisation / Dye } Tests
OR Toxoplasmin (skin) test (unreliable)

Pneumocystis carinii
Causing interstitial plasma cell pneumonia

Morphology
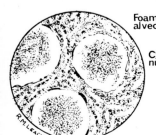
Foam-like masses in alveoli and bronchii
Cysts with up to 8 nuclei described (Special staining method)

Life cycle Unknown

Laboratory diagnosis Post mortem histology

Pathology
DISTENDED
THICK PLEURA
CUT SURFACE GREY
AIRLESS
SEPTAE THICK
MICRO.
Alveolar epithelium thick partly desquamated
Infiltration leucocytes and plasma cells
Exudate, inflammatory cells and pneumocystis carinii in lumen

PLATE 71

Recapitulation

Morphological differentiations

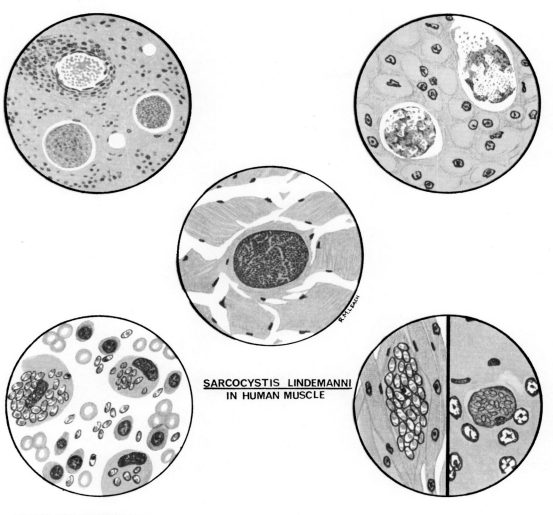

TOXOPLASMA IN PSEUDOCYSTS
IN VARIOUS CELLS

EXOERYTHROCYTIC SCHIZONTS OF PLASMODIUM
IN LIVER CELLS

SARCOCYSTIS LINDEMANNI
IN HUMAN MUSCLE

LEISHMAN DONOVAN BODIES IN
R.E. CELLS IN VISCERAL
LEISHMANIASIS

LEISHMANIAL FORMS OF TRYPANOSOMA CRUZI
IN MYOCARDIAL AND C.N.S. CELLS.

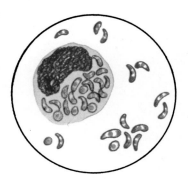

Toxoplasma gondii
NOT in blood

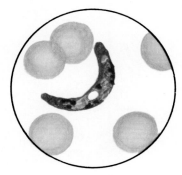

Ookinete of plasmodium
in mosquito's stomach

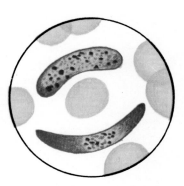

Gametocytes of P.falciparium
in blood

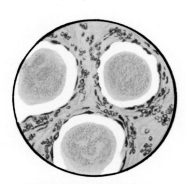

Pneumocystis carinii in lung

PLATE 72

Recapitulation

Protozoa inhabiting the intestine

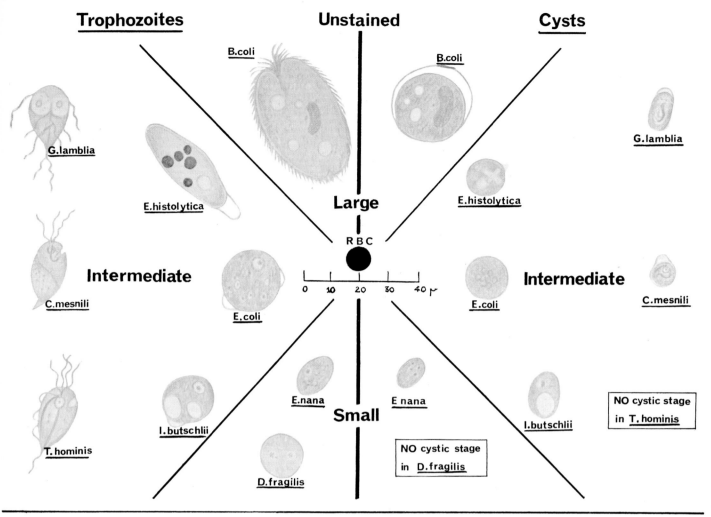

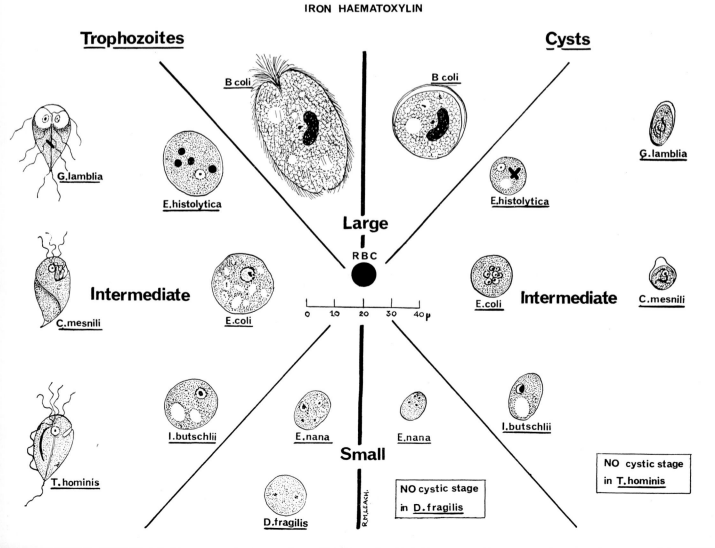

PART III

Further classification and morphology of worms of medical importance, with notes on the less common species.

CONTENTS

                                                                          PLATE

CESTODA   General morphology   73-74
                 Life cycle, in general   75
                 Classification   76
                 Pseudophyllidian tape worms of man   77
                        Genera and species   76
                        Dibothriocephalus latus   77
                        Diplogonoporous grandis   77
                        SPARGANOSIS   78
                 Cyclophyllidian tapeworms of man   79
                        Classification   79
                        Hymenolepis spp.   79
                        Taenia solium and Taenia saginata   80
                        Echinococcus granulosus and Echinococcus multilocularis 81
                        Multiceps (Taenia) multiceps   81
                        COENURUS CEREBRALIS   81
                        Inermicapsifer spp.   82
                        Bertiella studeri   82
                        Dipylidium caninum   82
                        Raillietina spp.   82

TREMATODA   General morphology and life cycle   83-84 and 85
                 Classification   86-87
                        Fasciola hepatica   88
                        Fasciola gigantica   88
                        Fasciolopsis buski   88
                        Dicrocoelium dendriticum   89
                        Clonorchis sinensis   89
                        Opisthorchis felineus   89
                        Heterophyes heterophyes   90
                        Metagonimus yokogawai   90
                        Paragonimus westermani   91
                        Echinostoma spp.   91
                        Gastrodiscoides hominis   91
                        Watsonius watsoni   91

NEMATODA   General morphology   92
                 Life cycle in general   93-94
                 Abridged classification   95-96
                 Aphasmid nematodes
                        Trichinella spiralis   97
                        Trichuris trichiura   97
                        Capillaria hepatica   97
                        Mermithid worms   98
                        Dioctophyma renale   98
                 Phasmid nematodes   98
                        Strongyloides stercoralis   98
                        HOOKWORMS.   Morphology   99
                               Ancylostoma duodenale   100
                               Ancylostoma braziliense   100
                               Ancylostoma caninum   100
                        Terniden deminutus   101
                        Oesophagostomum apiostomum   101
                        Syngamus laryngeus   101
                        Trichostrongylus spp.   102
                        Haemonchus contortus   102
                        Metastrongylus elongatus   102
                        Enterobius vermicularis   103
                        Ascaris lumbricoides   103
                        Toxicara canis and toxicara cati   104
                        Gongylonema pulchrum   104
                        Gnathostoma spinigerum   105 and 109
                        Physoloptera caucasica   105
                        Thelazia callipaeda   105

                 FILARIA WORMS

                        Wuchereria bancrofti   106
                        Brugia malayi   106
                        Onchocerca volvulus   106
                        Loa loa   106
                        Dipetalonema (acanthochielonema) perstans   106
                        Dipetalonema streptocerca   106
                        Mansonella ozzardi   107
                        Dirofilaria spp.   108
                        Dracunculus medinensis   108
                 LARVA MIGRANS.   Cutaneous   109
                                  Visceral.   110-111

MISCELLANEOUS WORMS
        GORDIACEA   112
        ACANTHOCEPHALA.
                Macrocanthorhynchus hirudinaceus   112
                Moniliformis moniliformis   112

RECAPITULATION
        Ova of the less common or less important worms   113
        Pathogenesis and pathology of worm infections   114
                Factors and general effects   115
                Local effects in general   115
                Particular local effects on:
                        The Brain and Spinal cord   116
                        The Eye   116
                        The Mouth and Pharynx   116
                        The Respiratory passages and Lungs   117
                        The Liver and Bile ducts   117
                        The Pancreas   117
                        The Intestinal tract   118
                        The Urinary tract   119
                        The Lymphatic System   119
                        The Circulatory System   120
                        The Skin and Subcutaneous tissue   121
                        The Muscle and Bone   121

Plate 73

Further classification and morphology of worms of medical importance, with notes on the less common species

INITIAL CLASSIFICATION (See plate 1 for details.)

Sub-kingdom   METAZOA

Phylum   PLATYHELMINTHES   NEMATHELMINTHES   Acanthocephala

Class   CESTODA   TREMATODA   NEMATODA   Nematophora

Cestoda (Tapeworms)

General Morphology

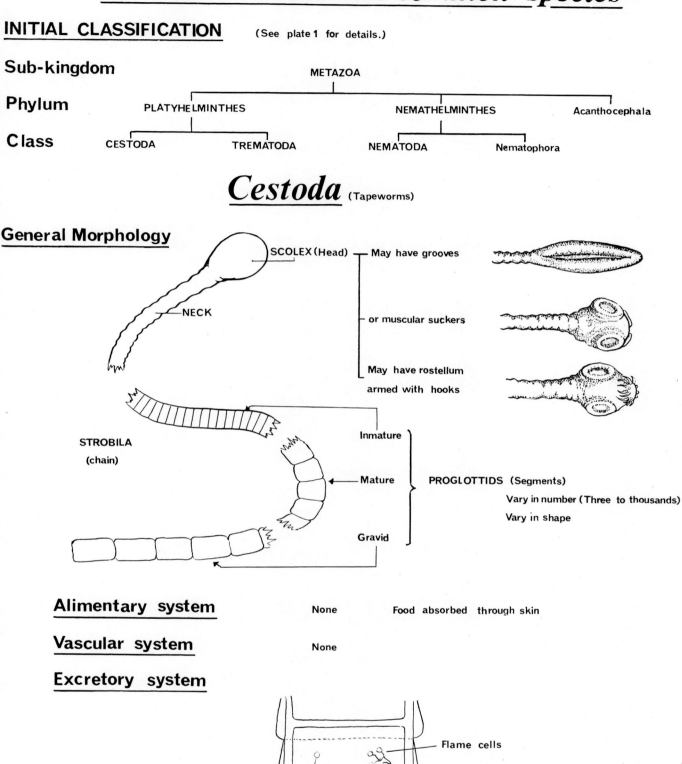

SCOLEX (Head) — May have grooves

— or muscular suckers

— May have rostellum armed with hooks

NECK

STROBILA (chain)

Inmature

Mature — PROGLOTTIDS (Segments)
Vary in number (Three to thousands)
Vary in shape

Gravid

Alimentary system

None   Food absorbed through skin

Vascular system

None

Excretory system

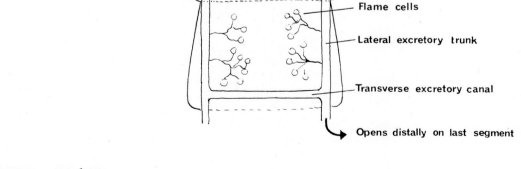

Flame cells

Lateral excretory trunk

Transverse excretory canal

Opens distally on last segment

Nervous system

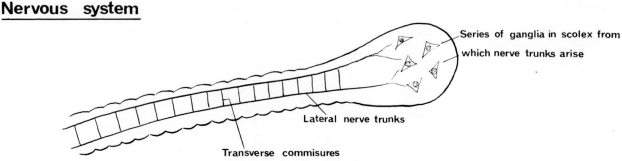

Series of ganglia in scolex from which nerve trunks arise

Lateral nerve trunks

Transverse commisures

Reproductive system

COMPLETE SET(S) OF ♂ AND ♀ ORGANS IN EACH PROGLOTTID

Common genital pore

May open :–

On ventral surface (with uterine pore) as in Dibothriocephalus

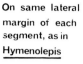

On same lateral margin of each segment, as in Hymenolepis

Testes

May be:–

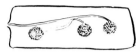

Few and large as in Hymenolepis

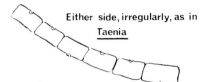

Either side, irregularly, as in Taenia

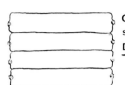

One on each side as in Diplogonoporus

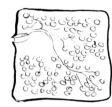

Numerous (500 or more) and small as in Taenia, Dibothriocephalus

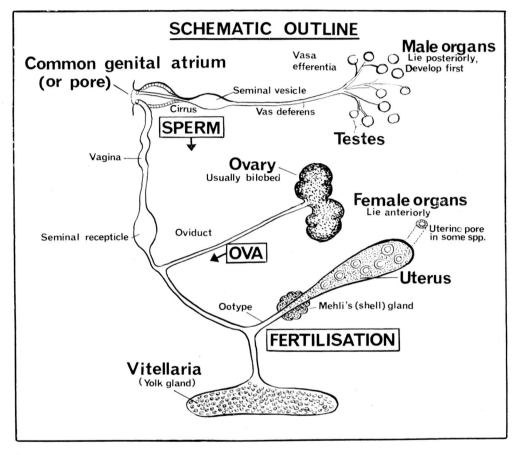

SCHEMATIC OUTLINE

Common genital atrium (or pore) — Vasa efferentia — **Male organs** Lie posteriorly, Develop first — Seminal vesicle — Cirrus — Vas deferens — **SPERM** — **Testes** — Vagina — Ovary Usually bilobed — **Female organs** Lie anteriorly — Seminal recepticle — Oviduct — **OVA** — Uterine pore in some spp. — **Uterus** — Ootype — Mehli's (shell) gland — **FERTILISATION** — Vitellaria (Yolk gland)

VITELLARIA May be:–

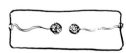

Single (for each set of genitalia) as in Dipylidium

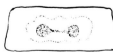

Bilobed (behind uterus) as in Hymenolepis

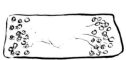

Numerous, small, scattered laterally as in Dibothriocephalus

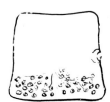

Numerous, small, scattered distally as in Taeniae

MATURE UTERUS May be:–

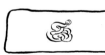

A coiled tube opening on surface as in Dibothriocephalus

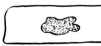

Saccular, as in Hymenolepis

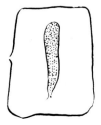

A central blind straight tube as in Taeniae

GRAVID UTERUS May be:–

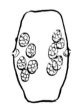

Reticular with ova in capsules, as in Dipylidium

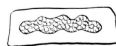

A lobular, transverse sac, as in Dipylidium

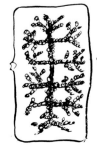

With lateral branches as in Taeniae

PLATE 75

Cestoda (Cont.)

LIFE CYCLE IN GENERAL.
1. NO INTERMEDIATE HOST REQUIRED - as in Hymenolepis nana

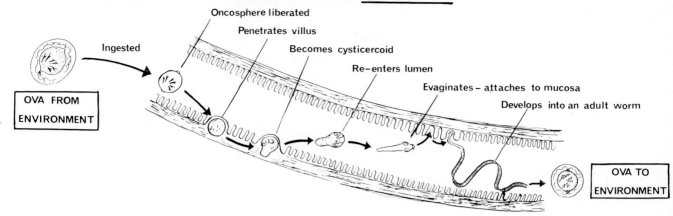

2. INTERMEDIATE HOST(S) REQUIRED - as in all other species of Cestoda.
A. Immature ova mature and hatch in water - as in Pseudophyllidea

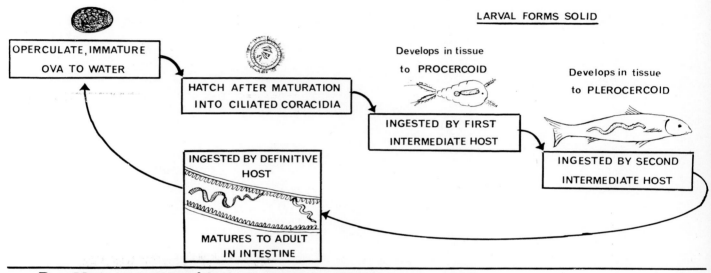

B. Mature ova voided to environment - as in Cyclophyllidea

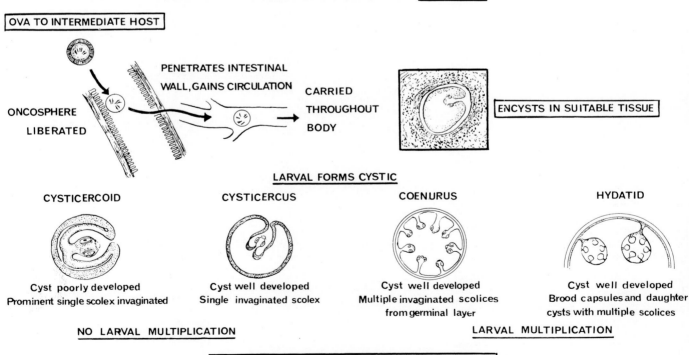

Plate 76

Cestoda (Cont.)

Classification.

	PSEUDOPHYLLIDEA		CYCLOPHYLLIDEA
ORDER			

2 sucking grooves	SCOLEX	4 muscular suckers
Centre of segment	GENITAL PORE	Margin(s) of segment
Centre of segment	UTERINE PORE	None. Uterus ends blindly
Coiled	UTERUS	Sac-like or Branched or Contains egg capsules
Operculate Immature	OVA	Non-operculate Mature
Ciliated (Coracidium)	ONCHOSPHERE	Non-ciliated 6-hooked
Procercoid Plerocercoid Larval forms SOLID	LARVAE	Cysticercoid Cysticercus Coenurus Hydatid Larval forms CYSTIC

PSEUDOPHYLLIDEAN TAPEWORMS OF MAN

GENUS.

DIBOTHRIOCEPHALUS

D. latus (and others)
Adult forms in man

D. mansonoides
(Sparganum mansoni)
Larval form in man

Adults unknown
(Sparganum proliferum)
Larval form in man.

Diplogonoporus

D. grandis
Adult form in man(rare)

PLATE 77

Cestoda. Pseudophyllidean tapeworms of man (Cont.)

DIBOTHRIOCEPHALUS LATUS
(The fish tape-worm)

Morphology

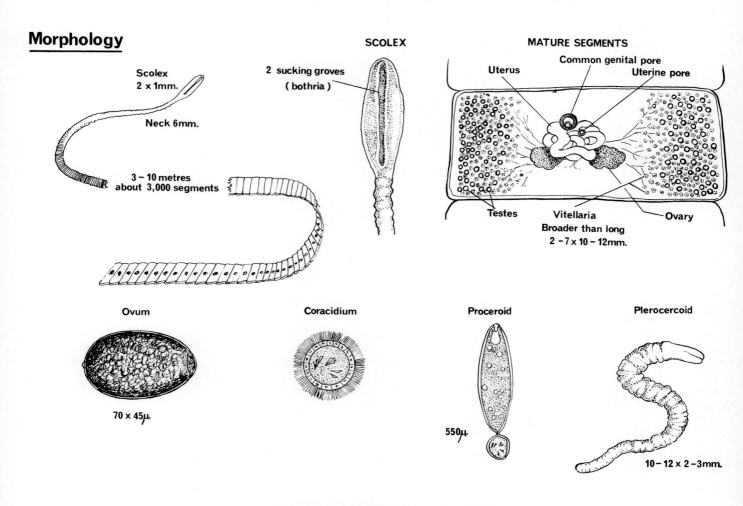

SCOLEX

MATURE SEGMENTS

Scolex
2 x 1mm.

Neck 6mm.

3 – 10 metres
about 3,000 segments

2 sucking groves
(bothria)

Uterus

Common genital pore

Uterine pore

Testes

Vitellaria
Broader than long
2 – 7 x 10 – 12mm.

Ovary

Ovum

Coracidium

Proceroid

Plerocercoid

70 x 45μ

550μ

10 – 12 x 2 –3mm.

LIFE CYCLE, PATHOLOGY, OCCURRENCE. – SEE PLATE 17

Diplogonoporus grandis

Morphology

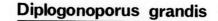

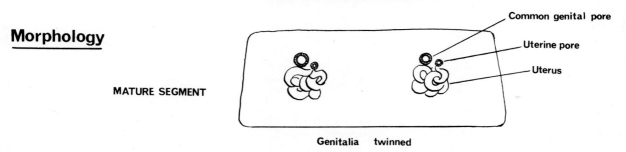

MATURE SEGMENT

Common genital pore

Uterine pore

Uterus

Genitalia   twinned

Life cycle

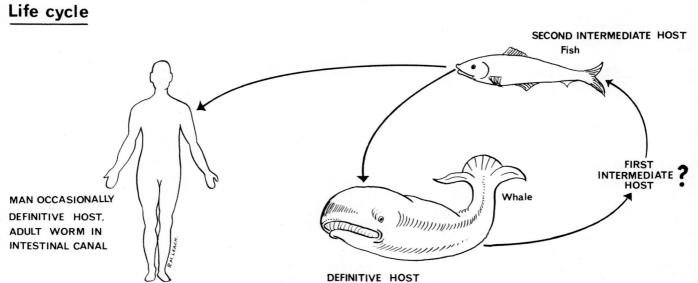

SECOND INTERMEDIATE HOST
Fish

MAN OCCASIONALLY
DEFINITIVE HOST.
ADULT WORM IN
INTESTINAL CANAL

Whale

FIRST
INTERMEDIATE
HOST ?

DEFINITIVE HOST

Occurrence – Reported 6 times in Japanese patients, causing intestinal upset.

Cestoda (Cont.)

PLATE 78

Larval forms of Pseudophyllidea in man
SPARGANOSIS

The extra-intestinal presence in human body of LARVAE of NON-human tapeworms of the genus DIBOTHRIOCEPHALUS

Life-cycle of such tapeworms

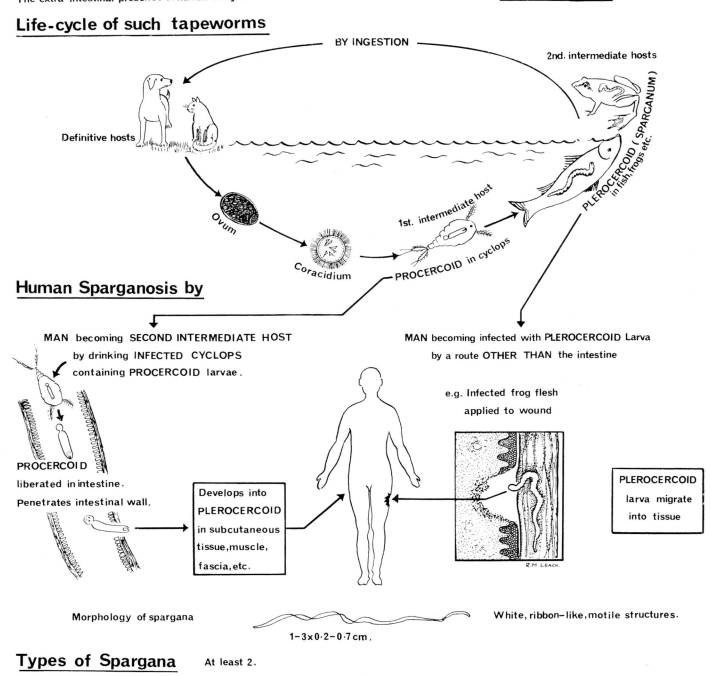

BY INGESTION

2nd. intermediate hosts

Definitive hosts

Ovum

Coracidium

1st. intermediate host

PROCERCOID in cyclops

PLEROCERCOID (SPARGANUM) in fish, frogs etc.

Human Sparganosis by

MAN becoming SECOND INTERMEDIATE HOST
by drinking INFECTED CYCLOPS
containing PROCERCOID larvae.

PROCERCOID
liberated in intestine.
Penetrates intestinal wall.

Develops into
PLEROCERCOID
in subcutaneous
tissue, muscle,
fascia, etc.

MAN becoming infected with PLEROCERCOID Larva
by a route OTHER THAN the intestine

e.g. Infected frog flesh
applied to wound

R.M LEACH.

PLEROCERCOID
larva migrate
into tissue

Morphology of spargana

$1-3 \times 0.2-0.7$ cm.

White, ribbon-like, motile structures.

Types of Spargana   At least 2.

1. Sparganum mansoni.   Plerocercoid stage of Dibothriocephalus mansonoides (dog and cat tapeworm)
    Does not proliferate in human tissues.

2. Sparganum proliferans.   Plerocercoid stage of tapeworms the adults of which are unknown
    This larva   proliferates in human tissues.

Geographical Distribution. Far East, occasionally elsewhere.

Pathology.
LIVING LARVAE - Painful, oedematous reaction.
DEAD LARVAE - Intense local inflammatory reaction
            Numerous eosinophils.
            Sometimes abscess formation.
        Ocular sparganosis (in soft tissues near eye)
            Severe damage may result.
PROLIFERATING LARVAE - Thousands may develop in same host

Laboratory diagnosis.
            Of the disease - examination of biopsy material.
            Of the sparganum - determined by feeding recovered larvae to cats and dogs
                and studying resulting adult form.

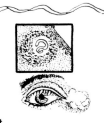

PLATE 79

Cestoda (Cont.)

Cyclophyllidean tapeworms of man

CLASSIFICATION

A. Of common or important occurrence

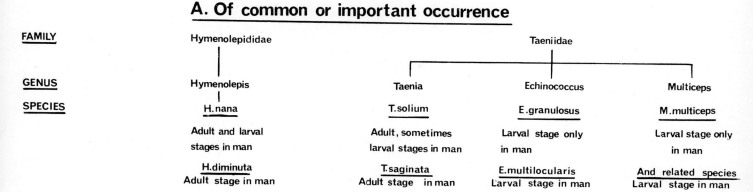

FAMILY	Hymenolepididae	Taeniidae		
GENUS	Hymenolepis	Taenia	Echinococcus	Multiceps
SPECIES	H.nana	T.solium	E.granulosus	M.multiceps
	Adult and larval stages in man	Adult, sometimes larval stages in man	Larval stage only in man	Larval stage only in man
	H.diminuta Adult stage in man	T.saginata Adult stage in man	E.multilocularis Larval stage in man	And related species Larval stage in man

B. Occasionally infect man

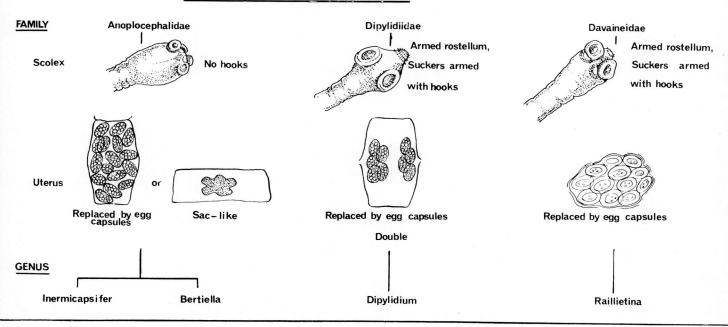

FAMILY — Anoplocephalidae — Dipylidiidae — Davaineidae

Scolex — No hooks — Armed rostellum, Suckers armed with hooks — Armed rostellum, Suckers armed with hooks

Uterus — Replaced by egg capsules   or   Sac–like — Replaced by egg capsules — Replaced by egg capsules

Double

GENUS — Inermicapsifer   Bertiella — Dipylidium — Raillietina

Dwarf tape-worms

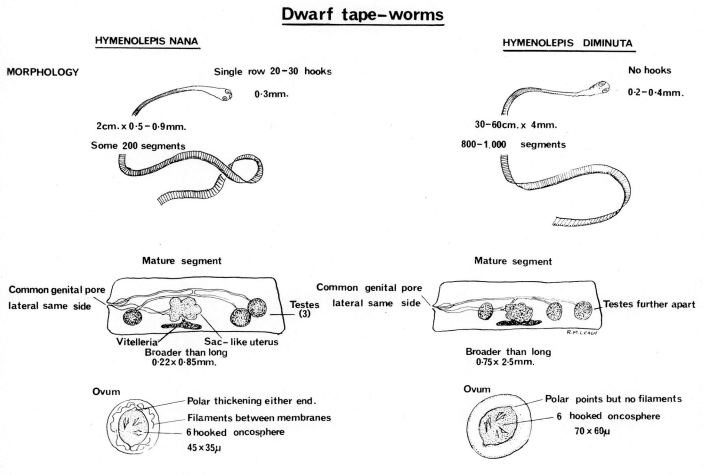

HYMENOLEPIS NANA

MORPHOLOGY

Single row 20–30 hooks
0·3mm.

2cm. x 0·5 – 0·9mm.

Some 200 segments

Mature segment

Common genital pore lateral same side

Testes (3)

Vitelleria   Sac – like uterus
Broader than long
0·22 x 0·85mm.

Ovum
— Polar thickening either end.
— Filaments between membranes
— 6 hooked oncosphere
45 x 35μ

HYMENOLEPIS DIMINUTA

No hooks
0·2 – 0·4mm.

30–60cm. x 4mm.

800–1,000   segments

Mature segment

Common genital pore lateral same side

Testes further apart

R.M.LEACH

Broader than long
0·75 x 2·5mm.

Ovum
— Polar points but no filaments
— 6 hooked oncosphere
70 x 60μ

Life cycle. Pathology. Occurrence. – See plate 16

Cyclophyllidean tapeworms of man

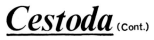

Taenia solium
(THE PORK TAPEWORM)

Taenia saginata
(THE BEEF TAPEWORM)

Morphology

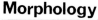

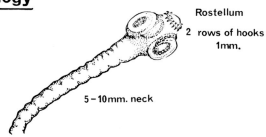

Rostellum
2 rows of hooks
1mm.

5 – 10 mm. neck

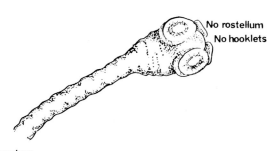

No rostellum
No hooklets

3 metres
800 – 1,000 segments

5 – 10 metres
1,000 – 2,000 segments

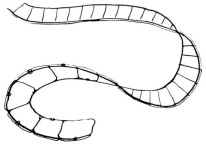

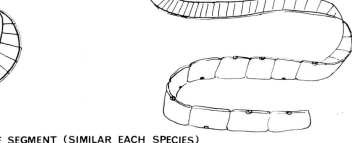

MATURE SEGMENT (SIMILAR EACH SPECIES)

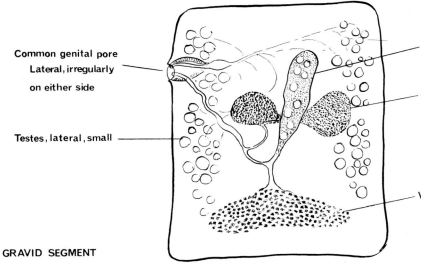

Common genital pore
Lateral, irregularly
on either side

Testes, lateral, small

Uterus, simple tube

Ovary, bilobed

Vitellaria, scattered, dorsal

GRAVID SEGMENT

Roughly square

GRAVID SEGMENT

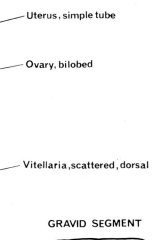

OVUM

(similar each species)

31 – 43 μ

Longer than broad
7 – 12 lateral uterine branches
12 × 6 mm.

Longer than broad
15 – 30 lateral uterine branches
16 – 20 × 5 – 7 mm.

CYSTICERCUS (larval form)

Cyst well developed

Invaginated scolex

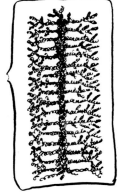

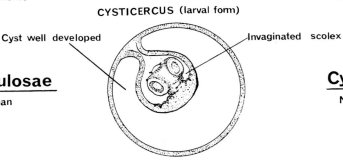

Cysticercus cellulosae
Occasionally found in man

Cysticercus bovis
Never found in man

Life Cycle, Pathology, Occurrence
See Plate 14

See Plate 15

PLATE 81

Cestoda (Cont.)

Cyclophyllidean tapeworms of man

Echinococcus granulosus and E. multilocularis

Larval stage (Hydatid and alveolar cysts) only in man.
See plates 18-19

Multiceps (or Taenia) multiceps

(The gid worm)

Larval stage only described in man, causing COENURUS CEREBRALIS

Life cycle

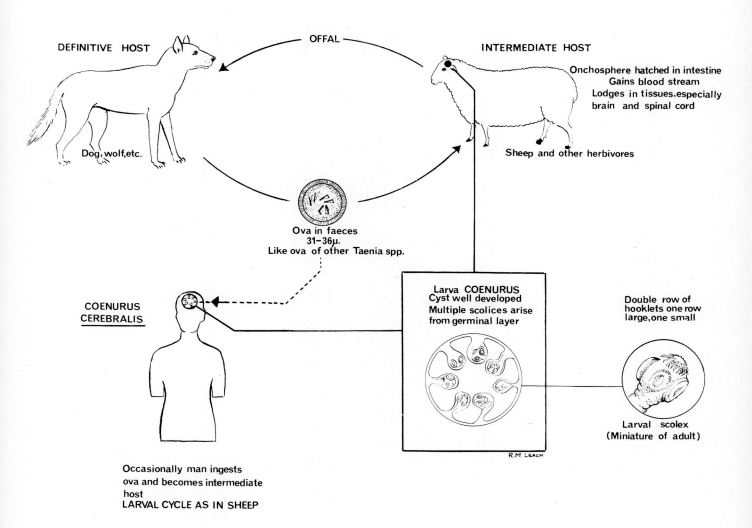

DEFINITIVE HOST

OFFAL

INTERMEDIATE HOST

Dog, wolf, etc.

Onchosphere hatched in intestine
Gains blood stream
Lodges in tissues, especially
brain and spinal cord

Sheep and other herbivores

Ova in faeces
31–36μ.
Like ova of other Taenia spp.

COENURUS
CEREBRALIS

Larva COENURUS
Cyst well developed
Multiple scolices arise
from germinal layer

Double row of
hooklets one row
large, one small

Larval scolex
(Miniature of adult)

R.M. LEACH

Occasionally man ingests
ova and becomes intermediate
host
LARVAL CYCLE AS IN SHEEP

Geographical distribution   Human cases scattered

Pathology   Space occupying lesion of brain or spinal cord

Laboratory diagnosis   Histological

Related species recorded as causing coenurus infection in man

SPECIES	DEFINITIVE HOST	INTERMEDIATE HOST USUALLY
Multiceps glomeratus	Unknown	Gerbille
M. serialis	Dogs, wolves, foxes	Rabbits and other rodents

PLATE 82

Cestoda (Cont.)

Cyclophyllidean tapeworms of man

Inermicapsifer spp.

Life cycle probably :

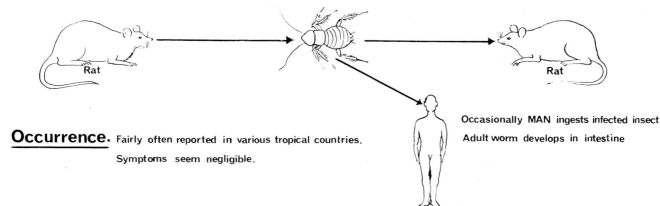

Arthropod e.g. cockroach

Rat

Rat

Occasionally MAN ingests infected insect

Adult worm develops in intestine

Occurrence. Fairly often reported in various tropical countries. Symptoms seem negligible.

Bertiella studeri.

Life cycle

Morphology of ovum distinctive

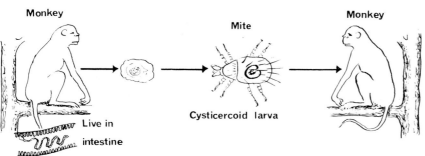

Monkey

Mite

Monkey

Cysticercoid larva

Live in intestine

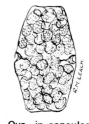

Irregular shape

Delicate middle membrane

Bicornuate protrusion of inner shell

$45 \times 50\,\mu$

Occurrence. Several human infections reported

Dipylidium caninum.

(The double-pored dog tapeworm)

Life cycle

Definitive host

Intermediate host

Morphology of gravid segment

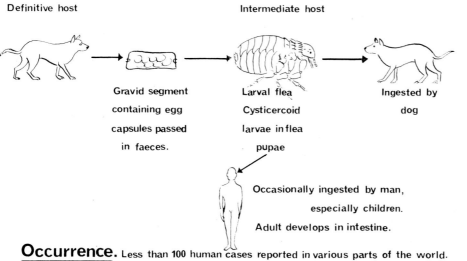

Gravid segment containing egg capsules passed in faeces.

Larval flea Cysticercoid larvae in flea pupae

Ingested by dog

Occasionally ingested by man, especially children.

Adult develops in intestine.

Ova in capsules Released when segment dries

OVUM

$25-40\mu$.

Occurrence. Less than 100 human cases reported in various parts of the world. Infection generally light with no symptoms or minor intestinal disturbance and toxic nervous manifestations in children.

Diagnosis. Segments or egg capsules in faeces.

Raillietina madagascarensis and other spp.

Life cycle. Not studied.

Occurrence. Occasionally adults found in man.

PLATE 83

Trematoda (Flukes)

GENERAL MORPHOLOGY AND LIFE CYCLE

A. Hermaphroditic spp. (All except genus Schistosoma)

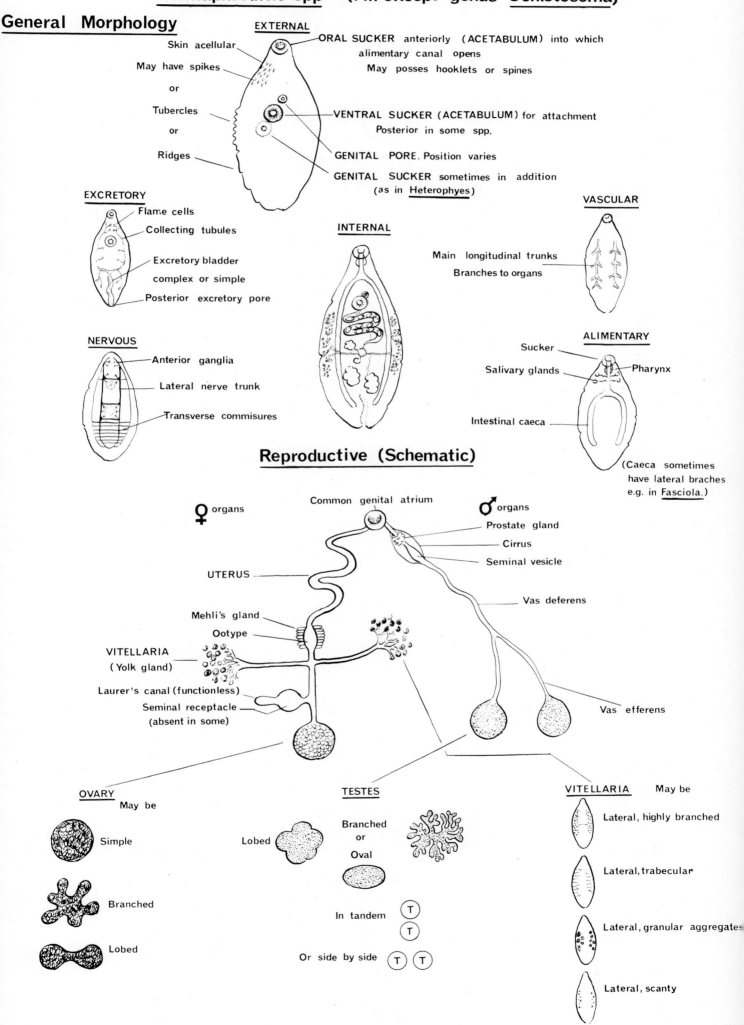

General Morphology

EXTERNAL

Skin acellular

May have spikes

or

Tubercles

or

Ridges

ORAL SUCKER anteriorly (ACETABULUM) into which
alimentary canal opens
May posses hooklets or spines

VENTRAL SUCKER (ACETABULUM) for attachment
Posterior in some spp.

GENITAL PORE. Position varies

GENITAL SUCKER sometimes in addition
(as in Heterophyes)

EXCRETORY
Flame cells
Collecting tubules
Excretory bladder
complex or simple
Posterior excretory pore

NERVOUS
Anterior ganglia
Lateral nerve trunk
Transverse commisures

INTERNAL

VASCULAR
Main longitudinal trunks
Branches to organs

ALIMENTARY
Sucker
Salivary glands
Pharynx
Intestinal caeca
(Caeca sometimes
have lateral braches
e.g. in Fasciola.)

Reproductive (Schematic)

♀ organs
Common genital atrium
♂ organs
Prostate gland
Cirrus
Seminal vesicle

UTERUS

Vas deferens

Mehli's gland
Ootype

VITELLARIA
(Yolk gland)

Laurer's canal (functionless)

Seminal receptacle
(absent in some)

Vas efferens

OVARY
May be
Simple
Branched
Lobed

TESTES
Lobed
Branched
or
Oval
In tandem
Or side by side

VITELLARIA
May be
Lateral, highly branched
Lateral, trabecular
Lateral, granular aggregates
Lateral, scanty

Life cycle in general

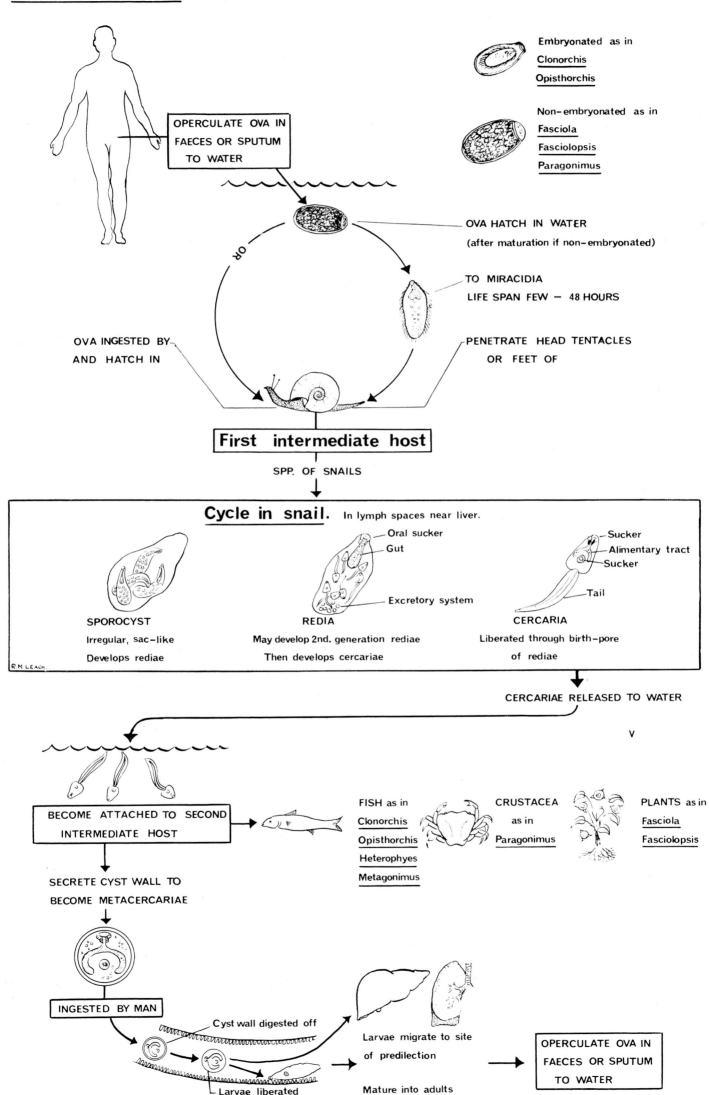

Embryonated as in
Clonorchis
Opisthorchis

Non-embryonated as in
Fasciola
Fasciolopsis
Paragonimus

OPERCULATE OVA IN
FAECES OR SPUTUM
TO WATER

OR

OVA HATCH IN WATER
(after maturation if non-embryonated)

TO MIRACIDIA
LIFE SPAN FEW — 48 HOURS

OVA INGESTED BY
AND HATCH IN

PENETRATE HEAD TENTACLES
OR FEET OF

First intermediate host

SPP. OF SNAILS

Cycle in snail. In lymph spaces near liver.

Oral sucker
Gut

Excretory system

Sucker
Alimentary tract
Sucker
Tail

SPOROCYST
Irregular, sac-like
Develops rediae

REDIA
May develop 2nd. generation rediae
Then develops cercariae

CERCARIA
Liberated through birth-pore
of rediae

R M LEACH

CERCARIAE RELEASED TO WATER

v

BECOME ATTACHED TO SECOND
INTERMEDIATE HOST

FISH as in
Clonorchis
Opisthorchis
Heterophyes
Metagonimus

CRUSTACEA
as in
Paragonimus

PLANTS as in
Fasciola
Fasciolopsis

SECRETE CYST WALL TO
BECOME METACERCARIAE

INGESTED BY MAN

Cyst wall digested off

Larvae migrate to site
of predilection

Mature into adults

Larvae liberated

OPERCULATE OVA IN
FAECES OR SPUTUM
TO WATER

B. Spp. with SEPARATE SEXES (Schistosoma spp.)

General morphology

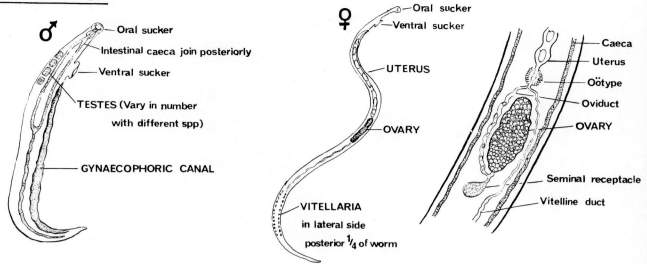

♂
- Oral sucker
- Intestinal caeca join posteriorly
- Ventral sucker
- TESTES (Vary in number with different spp)
- GYNAECOPHORIC CANAL

♀
- Oral sucker
- Ventral sucker
- UTERUS
- OVARY
- VITELLARIA in lateral side posterior ¼ of worm

- Caeca
- Uterus
- Oötype
- Oviduct
- OVARY
- Seminal receptacle
- Vitelline duct

Life cycle in general

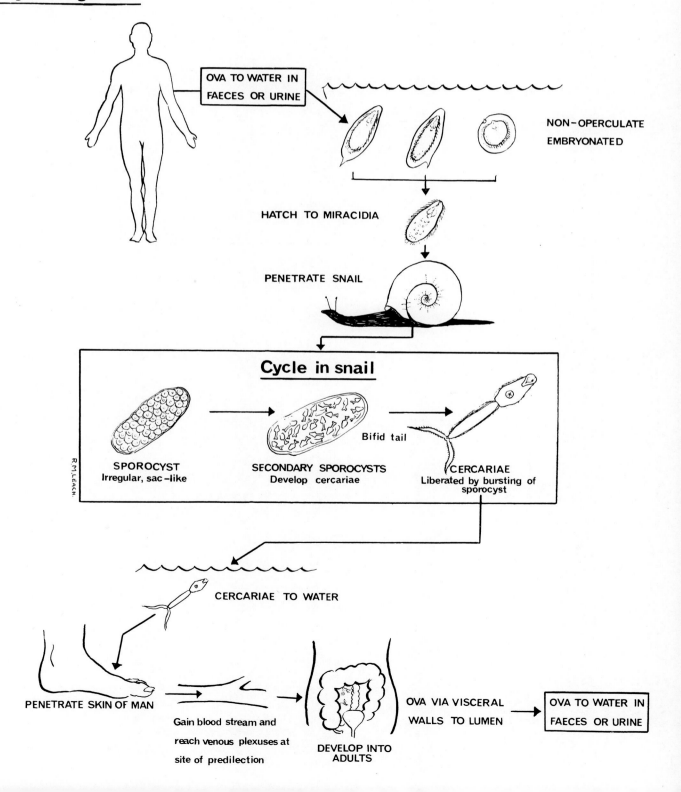

OVA TO WATER IN FAECES OR URINE

NON-OPERCULATE EMBRYONATED

HATCH TO MIRACIDIA

PENETRATE SNAIL

Cycle in snail

SPOROCYST
Irregular, sac-like

SECONDARY SPOROCYSTS
Develop cercariae

Bifid tail

CERCARIAE
Liberated by bursting of sporocyst

R.M.LEACH.

CERCARIAE TO WATER

PENETRATE SKIN OF MAN

Gain blood stream and reach venous plexuses at site of predilection

DEVELOP INTO ADULTS

OVA VIA VISCERAL WALLS TO LUMEN

OVA TO WATER IN FAECES OR URINE

Trematoda (Cont.)

PLATE 86

FURTHER CLASSIFICATION (Of those species affecting man)

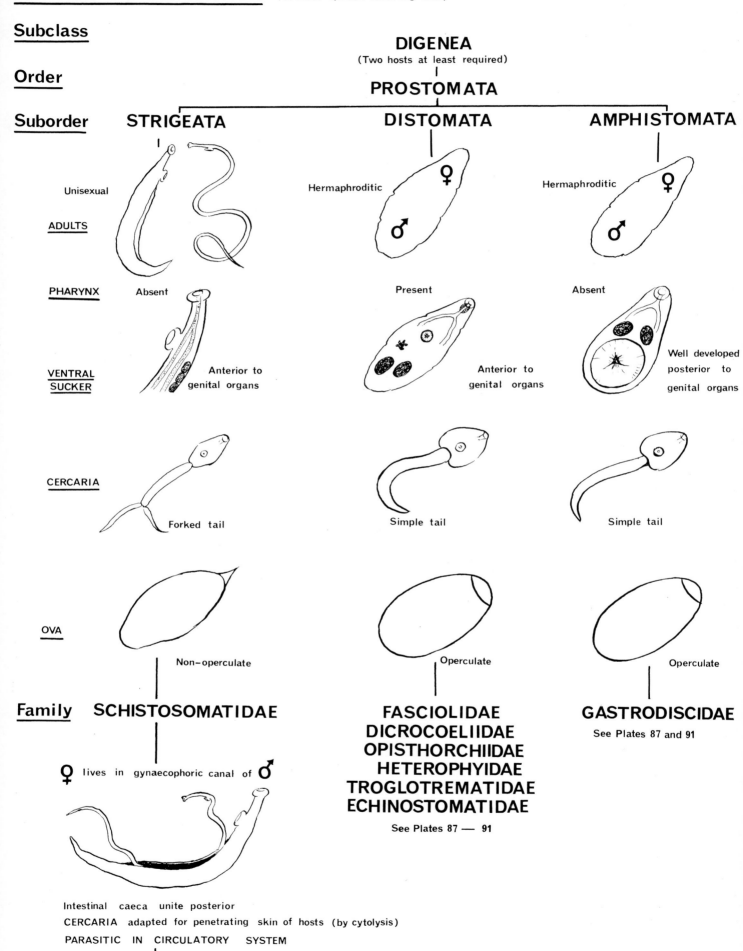

Subclass

DIGENEA
(Two hosts at least required)

Order

PROSTOMATA

Suborder

STRIGEATA   DISTOMATA   AMPHISTOMATA

Unisexual   Hermaphroditic   Hermaphroditic

ADULTS

PHARYNX   Absent   Present   Absent

VENTRAL SUCKER   Anterior to genital organs   Anterior to genital organs   Well developed posterior to genital organs

CERCARIA   Forked tail   Simple tail   Simple tail

OVA   Non-operculate   Operculate   Operculate

Family   SCHISTOSOMATIDAE   FASCIOLIDAE
DICROCOELIIDAE
OPISTHORCHIIDAE
HETEROPHYIDAE
TROGLOTREMATIDAE
ECHINOSTOMATIDAE

See Plates 87 — 91

GASTRODISCIDAE

See Plates 87 and 91

♀ lives in gynaecophoric canal of ♂

Intestinal caeca unite posterior
CERCARIA adapted for penetrating skin of hosts (by cytolysis)
PARASITIC IN CIRCULATORY SYSTEM

Genus   SCHISTOSOMA

Species   S.haematobium   See Plates 20 – 21
S.mansoni
S.japonicum

Plate 87

Trematoda, Classification (Cont.)

SUBORDER

DISTOMATA (See plate 86)

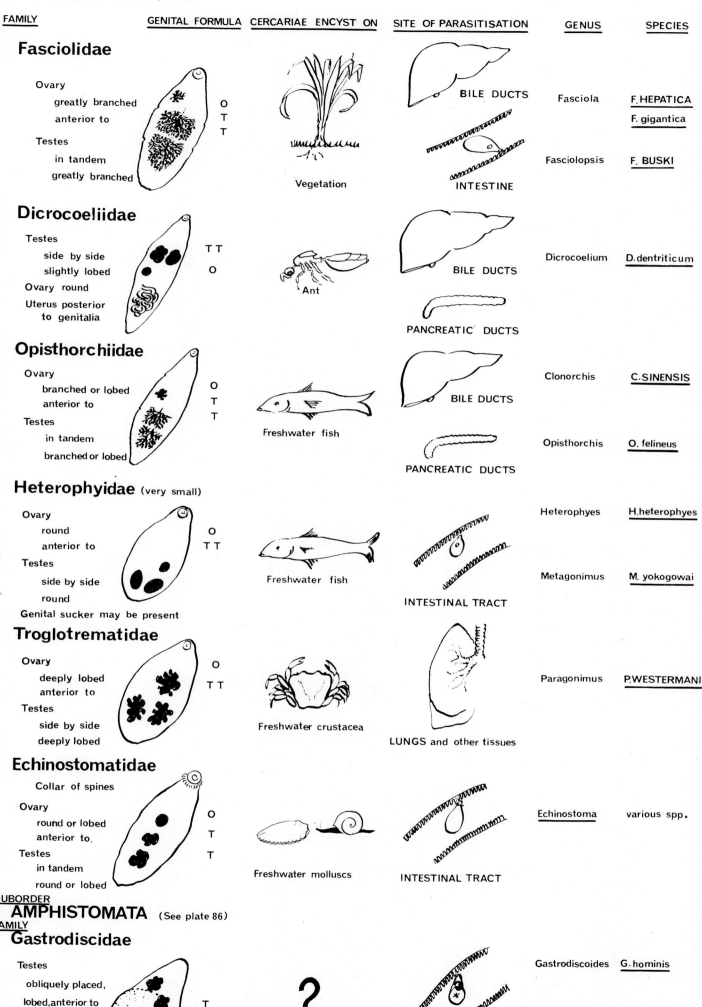

FAMILY	GENITAL FORMULA	CERCARIAE ENCYST ON	SITE OF PARASITISATION	GENUS	SPECIES

Fasciolidae

Ovary
greatly branched
anterior to
Testes
in tandem
greatly branched

O T T

Vegetation

BILE DUCTS — Fasciola — F. HEPATICA, F. gigantica

INTESTINE — Fasciolopsis — F. BUSKI

Dicrocoeliidae

Testes
side by side
slightly lobed
Ovary round
Uterus posterior
to genitalia

T T O

Ant

BILE DUCTS
PANCREATIC DUCTS — Dicrocoelium — D. dentriticum

Opisthorchiidae

Ovary
branched or lobed
anterior to
Testes
in tandem
branched or lobed

O T T

Freshwater fish

BILE DUCTS — Clonorchis — C. SINENSIS

PANCREATIC DUCTS — Opisthorchis — O. felineus

Heterophyidae (very small)

Ovary
round
anterior to
Testes
side by side
round
Genital sucker may be present

O T T

Freshwater fish

INTESTINAL TRACT — Heterophyes — H. heterophyes / Metagonimus — M. yokogowai

Troglotrematidae

Ovary
deeply lobed
anterior to
Testes
side by side
deeply lobed

O T T

Freshwater crustacea

LUNGS and other tissues — Paragonimus — P. WESTERMANI

Echinostomatidae

Collar of spines
Ovary
round or lobed
anterior to
Testes
in tandem
round or lobed

O T T

Freshwater molluscs

INTESTINAL TRACT — Echinostoma — various spp.

SUBORDER

AMPHISTOMATA (See plate 86)

FAMILY

Gastrodiscidae

Testes
obliquely placed,
lobed, anterior to
Ovary
lobed
Large ventral sucker posteriorly

T T O

?

INTESTINAL TRACT — Gastrodiscoides — G. hominis / Watsonius — W. watsoni

Trematoda (cont.)

PLATE 88

FAMILY **FASCIOLIDAE**

Fasciola hepatica

(The sheep liver fluke)

MORPHOLOGY

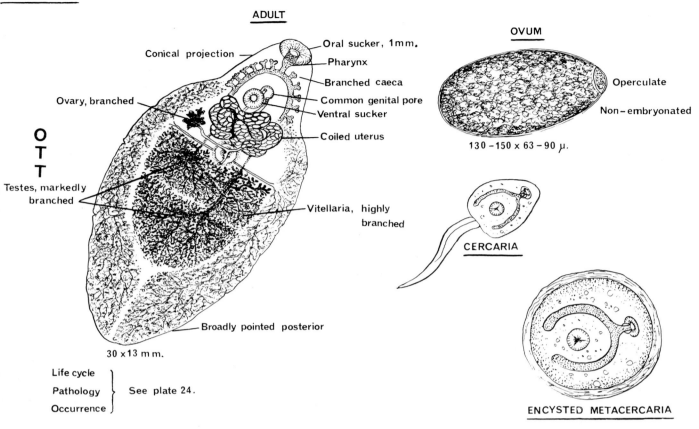

ADULT

Conical projection — Oral sucker, 1mm.
Pharynx
Branched caeca
Ovary, branched — Common genital pore
Ventral sucker
Coiled uterus

OTT

Testes, markedly branched

Vitellaria, highly branched

Broadly pointed posterior

30 x 13 mm.

OVUM

Operculate
Non–embryonated

130 – 150 x 63 – 90 μ.

CERCARIA

ENCYSTED METACERCARIA

Life cycle
Pathology } See plate 24.
Occurrence

Fasciola gigantica

(The giant liver fluke)

Similar to F.hepatica   somewhat larger eggs.   160 – 190 × 70 – 90 μ.

Occurrence   In herbivores in Africa and Far East.

Occasionally described in man.

Fasciolopsis buski

(The large intestinal fluke)

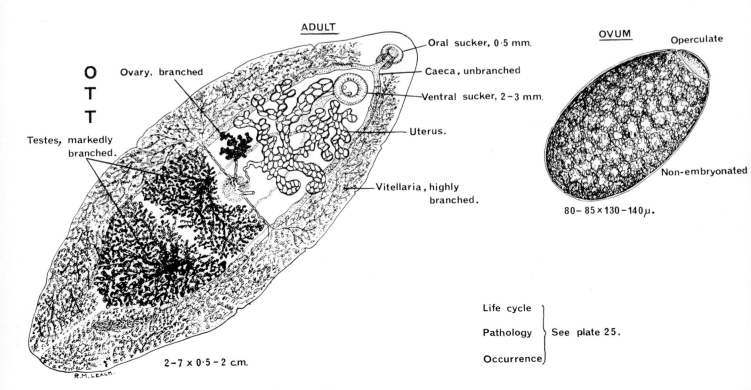

ADULT

Oral sucker, 0·5 mm.
Caeca, unbranched
Ovary, branched — Ventral sucker, 2–3 mm.
Uterus.

OTT

Testes, markedly branched.

Vitellaria, highly branched.

2 – 7 × 0·5 – 2 c.m.

R.M.LEACH.

OVUM

Operculate
Non–embryonated

80 – 85 × 130 – 140μ.

Life cycle
Pathology } See plate 25.
Occurrence

FAMILY DICROCOELIIDAE
Dicrocoelium dentriticum
(THE LANCET FLUKE)

Morphology

ADULT

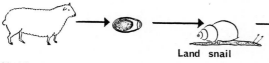

Testes slightly lobed
TT
O
Ovary round

Oral sucker
Caeca
Ventral sucker

Vitellaria scanty
Uterus coiled posterior

Lancet shaped, 5–14x1·5–2·5mm.

OVUM

Operculate
Embryonated

38–45×22–30μ.

CERCARIA

Stylet or oral sucker
Simple tail

700×70μ.

Life cycle

DEFINITIVE HOST   1st. INTERMEDIATE HOST   2nd. INTERMEDIATE HOST   DEFINITIVE HOST

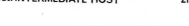

Land snail

?

Herbivores
Adult fluke in biliary passages

Occasionally man ingests infected ants and harbours adult worms

Spurious infections (eggs in faeces) from eating liver infected by adult worms

Occurrence   A few scattered human infections recorded
Pathology like <u>F. hepatica</u>, less marked

FAMILY Opisthorchiidae
Clonorchis sinensis
(THE CHINESE LIVER FLUKE)

ADULT

Morphology

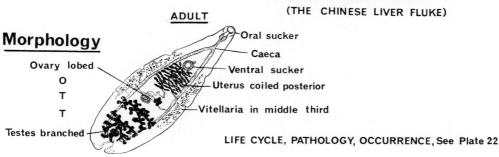

Ovary lobed
O
T
T
Testes branched

Oral sucker
Caeca
Ventral sucker
Uterus coiled posterior
Vitellaria in middle third

LIFE CYCLE, PATHOLOGY, OCCURRENCE, See Plate 22

10–20mm. x 3–4 mm.

OVUM

Operculate embryonated

29 x 16μ.

CERCARIA

Conspicuous eye spots

Opisthorchis felineus
(THE CAT LIVER FLUKE)

Morphology

ADULT

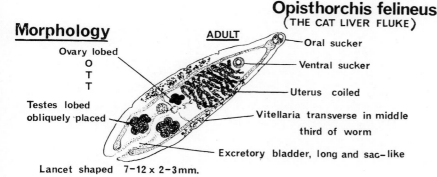

Ovary lobed
O
T
T
Testes lobed obliquely placed

Oral sucker
Ventral sucker
Uterus coiled
Vitellaria transverse in middle third of worm
Excretory bladder, long and sac–like

Lancet shaped 7–12 x 2–3mm.

OVUM

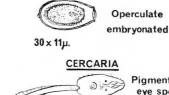

Operculate embryonated

30 x 11μ.

CERCARIA

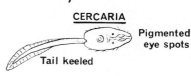

Pigmented eye spots
Tail keeled

Life cycle

DEFINITIVE HOST

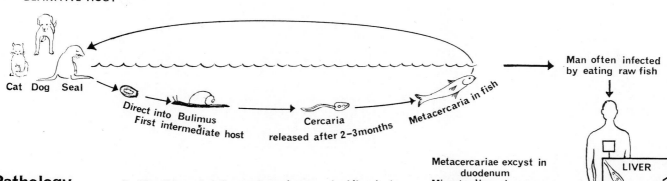

Cat Dog Seal

Direct into Bulimus
First intermediate host

Cercaria released after 2–3months

Metacercaria in fish

Man often infected by eating raw fish

Metacercariae excyst in duodenum
Migrate through common bile duct to distal bile passages
Mature in 3–4 weeks

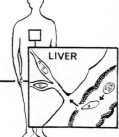

LIVER

Pathology   Proliferative and inflammatory changes in bile ducts.
Cirrhosis if massive or repeated infection

Occurrence   Mainly Eastern Europe and Russia

R.M. LEACH.

Plate 90

Trematoda (cont.)
Family   HETEROPHYIDAE
Heterophyes heterophyes

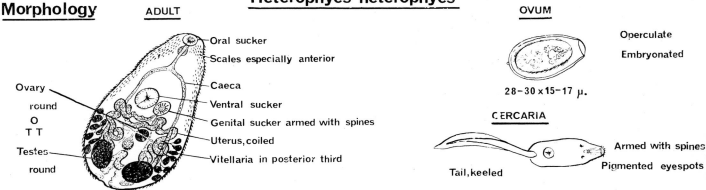

Morphology

ADULT

- Oral sucker
- Scales especially anterior
- Caeca
- Ventral sucker
- Genital sucker armed with spines
- Uterus, coiled
- Vitellaria in posterior third

Ovary
round
O
T T
Testes
round

Very small 1–1.7 × 0.3–0.4 mm.

OVUM

Operculate
Embryonated

28–30 × 15–17 μ.

CERCARIA

Armed with spines
Pigmented eyespots
Tail, keeled

Life cycle

Definitive hosts

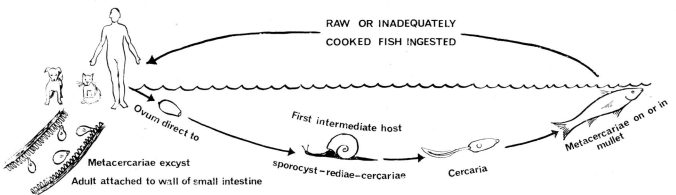

RAW OR INADEQUATELY
COOKED FISH INGESTED

Ovum direct to

First intermediate host

sporocyst – rediae – cercariae

Cercaria

Metacercariae on or in mullet

Metacercariae excyst

Adult attached to wall of small intestine

Pathology

Mild inflammatory reaction.
Ectopic ova reported in heart and brain

Occurrence

Nile delta; Far East.

Metagonimus yokogawai

Morphology

ADULT

- Oral sucker
- Pharynx
- Caeca
- Ventral sucker
- Uterus coiled
- Conspicuous seminal receptacle

Ovary
round
O
T T
Testes
round

Very small (one of smallest human flukes) 1.5 × 0.6 mm.

OVUM

Operculate
Embryonated

27 × 16 μ. (like Heterophyes)

CERCARIA (like Heterophyes)

Spines
Eyespots
Tail keeled

Life cycle

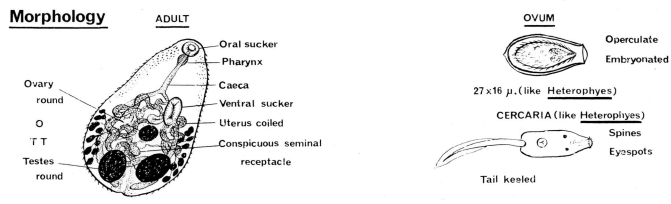

Definitive hosts

UNCOOKED FISH

Ovum direct to

sporocyst – rediae – cercariae

Cercariae

Metacercariae in fish

Adult in small intestine

Occurrence

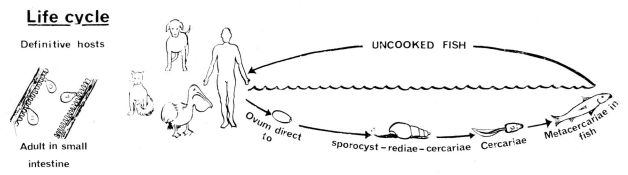

Prevalent in Far East and parts of Central Europe.
Causes mild inflammatory reaction in intestine.
Occasionally ectopic ova cause granulomata in other organs
especially liver and brain.

OTHER SPECIES OF **Metagonimus.**

Closely related species have been described occasionally.
Ectopic ova in men may cause variety of syndromes
especially cardiac like beri beri and cerebral
haemorrhage.

PLATE 91

Trematoda (Cont.)
Family TROGLOTREMATIDAE
PARAGONIMUS WESTERMANI

Morphology

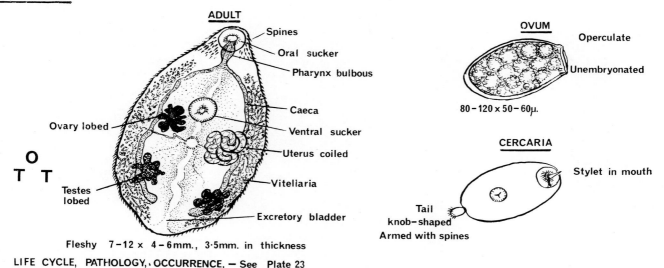

ADULT

Spines
Oral sucker
Pharynx bulbous
Caeca
Ventral sucker
Ovary lobed
Uterus coiled
O
T T
Testes lobed
Vitellaria
Excretory bladder

Fleshy 7−12 x 4−6mm., 3·5mm. in thickness

LIFE CYCLE, PATHOLOGY, OCCURRENCE, − See Plate 23

OVUM
Operculate
Unembryonated
80 − 120 x 50 − 60μ.

CERCARIA
Stylet in mouth
Tail knob−shaped
Armed with spines

Family ECHINOSTOMATIDAE
Echinostoma species

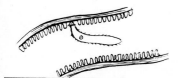

Intestinal flukes found in indigenous populations particularly in the Far East as common or occasional infections.
Relatively unimportant, but ova may be passed in faeces and require identification, mainly based on size.

Family GASTRODISCIDIAE
Gastrodiscoides hominis

Morphology

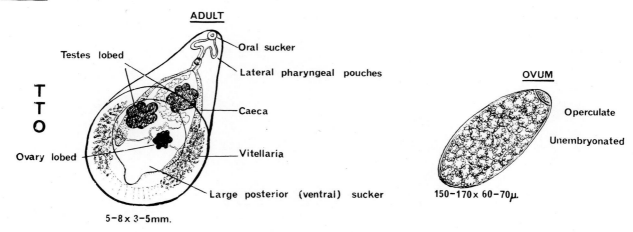

ADULT

Oral sucker
Testes lobed
Lateral pharyngeal pouches
T T O
Caeca
Ovary lobed
Vitellaria
Large posterior (ventral) sucker

5−8 x 3−5mm.

OVUM
Operculate
Unembryonated
150−170 x 60−70μ.

Life Cycle

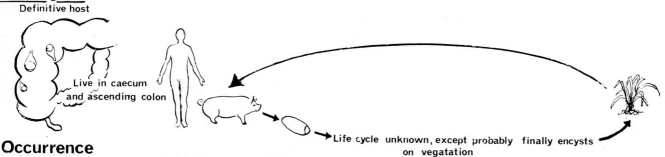

Definitive host
Live in caecum and ascending colon
Life cycle unknown, except probably finally encysts on vegatation

Occurrence

In man,(especially children),Assam, Bengal, Malaya. May cause mucosal inflammation.

Watsonius watsoni

A somewhat similar fluke occurs in the bowel of monkeys. One human case recorded.

Nematoda
(Round worms)

PLATE 92

General morphology

Long, cylindrical, unsegmented, generally tapering at each end.
Possess a body cavity and alimentary tract.
Sexes generally separate.

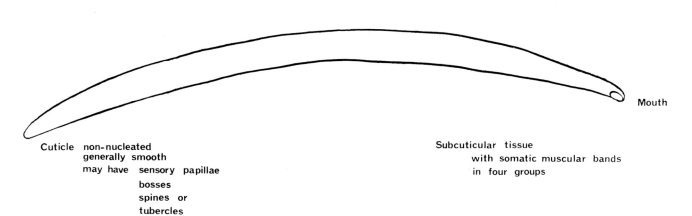

Mouth

Cuticle non-nucleated
generally smooth
may have sensory papillae
bosses
spines or
tubercles

Subcuticular tissue
with somatic muscular bands
in four groups

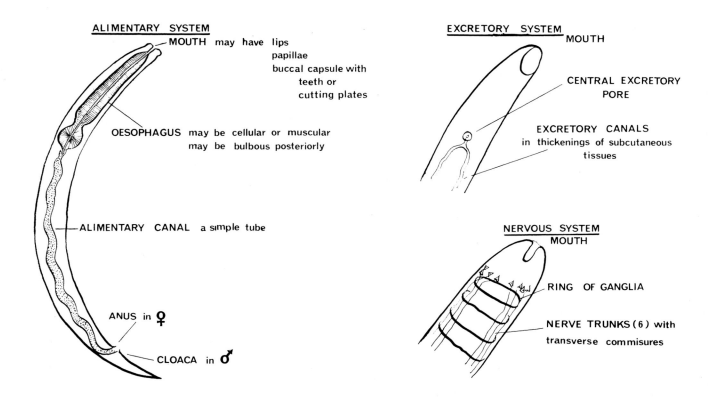

ALIMENTARY SYSTEM

MOUTH may have lips
papillae
buccal capsule with
teeth or
cutting plates

OESOPHAGUS may be cellular or muscular
may be bulbous posteriorly

ALIMENTARY CANAL a simple tube

ANUS in ♀

CLOACA in ♂

EXCRETORY SYSTEM

MOUTH

CENTRAL EXCRETORY
PORE

EXCRETORY CANALS
in thickenings of subcutaneous
tissue

NERVOUS SYSTEM

MOUTH

RING OF GANGLIA

NERVE TRUNKS (6) with
transverse commisures

Reproductive system

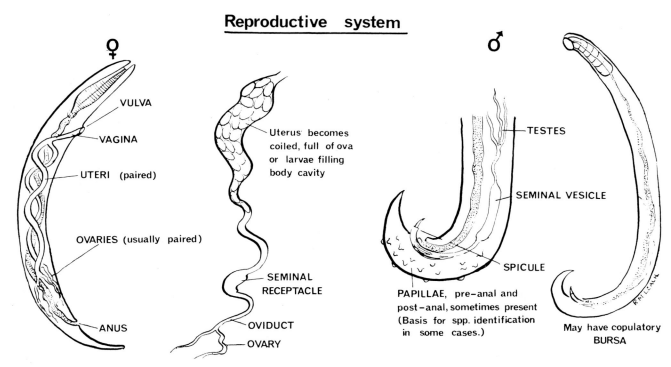

♀

VULVA

VAGINA

UTERI (paired)

OVARIES (usually paired)

ANUS

Uterus becomes
coiled, full of ova
or larvae filling
body cavity

SEMINAL
RECEPTACLE

OVIDUCT

OVARY

♂

TESTES

SEMINAL VESICLE

SPICULE

PAPILLAE, pre-anal and
post-anal, sometimes present
(Basis for spp. identification
in some cases.)

May have copulatory
BURSA

Plate 93

Nematoda (Cont.)

Life cycle in general

A. NO INTERMEDIATE HOST REQUIRED

OUTSIDE MAN	INFECTION BY	INSIDE MAN	SPECIES
EMBRYONATED OVA TO ENVIRONEMT	INGESTION	DEVELOP TO ADULT IN INTESTINE	Enterobius vermicularis
NON-EMBRYONATED OVA TO ENVIRONMENT		DEVELOP TO ADULT IN INTESTINE	Trichuris trichiura
MATURE IN DAMP SOIL	INGESTION	LARVAL CYCLE — Lung → Respiratory tree → Oesophagus; Blood; Ova hatch; Develop to adult in intestine	Ascaris lumbricoides / Toxocara spp. in animals. Larval stage only in man
MATURE, HATCH, ENCYST ON VEGETATION	INGESTION ENCYSTED	DEVELOP TO ADULT IN INTESTINE	Trichostrongylus spp / Haemonchus contortus
MATURE AND HATCH IN DAMP SOIL	PIERCING SKIN	LARVAL CYCLE — Blood; Skin; Develop to adult in intestine	Hookworms i.e. Ancylostoma duodenale / A. braziliense (human strains) / Necator americanus
OVA LAID IN TISSUES — IN LIVER	INGESTION OF INFECTED TISSUE	INTESTINE TO LIVER	Capillaria hepatica
IN INTESTINAL WALL — LARVAE TO GUT LUMEN; LARVAE RE-ENTER HOST; LARVAE TO ENVIRONMENT; INFECT NEW HOST; BECOME FREE LIVING; LARVAE FROM FREE CYCLE	PIERCING MUCOSA OR ANAL SKIN; PIERCING SKIN; PIERCING SKIN	LARVAL CYCLE — Blood; Develop to adult in intestine	Strongyloides stercoralis

B. INTERMEDIATE HOST(S) REQUIRED

OUTSIDE MAN	INTERMEDIATE HOST	INFECTION OF MAN BY	INSIDE MAN	
EMBRYONATED OVA TO ENVIRONMENT	INGESTED BY BEETLES — LARVAE HATCH AND ENCYST	INGESTION OF INFECTED BEETLES	INTESTINE TO BUCCAL CAVITY	Gongylonema pulchrum
HATCH IN SOIL	INGESTED BY EARTHWORMS	INGESTION OF EARTHWORMS	INTESTINE TO LUNGS	Metastrongylus elongatus

R.M.LEACH.

PLATE 94

Nematoda (Cont.)

Life cycle in general: B, Intermediate host(s) required, continued.

OUTSIDE MAN	INTERMEDIATE HOST	INFECTION OF MAN BY	INSIDE, MAN OR OTHER HOST	SPECIES
NON – EMBRYONATED OVA TO ENVIRONMENT	Ingested by leech Larvae developed Ingested by	Ingestion of fish	Intestine to Renal pelvis	Dioctophyma renale
Mature and hatch in damp soil	Ingested by Cyclops Larvae develop Cyclops ingested by Fish Frogs Snakes	Ingestion of infected flesh	Mature in stomach wall	Gnathostoma spinigerum Larval stage only in man
LARVIPAROUS In blood or tissue juices	Ingested by Insects Cyclical development	Bite of insect	Mature in lymph vessels Subcutaneous tissue	Filarial worms Wuchereria bancrofti Brugia malayi Loa loa Onchocerca volvulus
Through skin to water	Ingested by Cyclops	Ingestion of cyclops	Retroperitoneal then subcutaneous tissue	Dracunculus medinensis
In bowel wall	Via Blood to Muscle same host	Ingestion of Infected muscle	Mature in bowel, larviposit in wall	Trichinella spiralis

C,   Life cycle obscure

OUTSIDE MAN	CONJECTURAL CYCLE	INSIDE MAN AND OTHER HOSTS	
EMBRYONATED OVA TO ENVIRONMENT	Beetles 2nd. Intermediate host Fly	Matures in intestine Matures in conjunctiva	Physaloptera caucasia Thelazia callipaeda
NON - EMBRYONATED OVA TO ENVIRONMENT	Matures and hatches in soil larvae swallowed	Matures in intestine Matures in wall of caecum then in lumen	Ternidens deminutus Oesophagostomum apiostomum
	? Earthworm	Matures in respiratory passage	Syngamus laryngeus

PLATE 95

Nematoda (Cont.)

ABRIDGED CLASSIFICATION

CLASS: **APHASMIDIA** — NO CAUDAL CHEMO-RECEPTOR ORGANS **PHASMIDIA** — WITH CAUDAL CHEMO-RECEPTOR ORGANS

APHASMID NEMATODES

Superfamily	Size & shape	Mouth & oesophagus	Tail in ♂	Reproduction	Genus	Species
TRICHINELLOIDEA	Small, delicate, may be attenuated anteriorly.	No buccal capsule, oesophagus degenerate.	No bursa	Larviparous or oviparous	TRICHINELLA	SPIRALIS
					TRICHURIS	TRICHURA
					Capillaria	hepatica
MERMITHOIDEA	Long, pointed anteriorly	Non-muscular oesophagus		Oviparous	Spurious infections in man	
DICOTOPHYMATOIDEA	Large, attenuated ends	No buccal capsule	Bursa present	Oviparous	Dioctophyma	renale

PHASMID NEMATODES

Superfamily	Size & shape	Mouth & oesophagus	Tail in ♂	Reproduction	Genus	Species
RHABDITOIDEA	Parasitic ♀ thin, ♂ stout	No buccal capsule. Oesophagus filariform in ♀, muscular bulbous in ♂	No bursa	Larviparous	STRONGYLOIDES	STERCORALIS
STRONGYLOIDEA	Small, delicate	Well developed buccal capsule	Bursa with rays present	Oviparous	ANCYLOSTOMA	DUODENALE
NOTE: does NOT include the genus STRONGYLOIDES, see above.					Ancylostoma	braziliense
					Ancylostoma	caninum
					NECATOR	AMERICANUS
					Ternidens	deminutis
					Oesophagostomum	apiostomum
					Syngamus	laryngeus
TRICHOSTRONGYLOIDEA	Small, slender	Capsule rudimentary or absent	Conspicuous bursa	Oviparous	Trichostrongylus	spp.
					Haemonchus	contortus
METASTRONGYLOIDEA	Small, filiform	Capsule rudimentary or absent. Pair of lateral tri-lobed lips	Bursa present, rays striated	Oviparous	Metastrongylus	elongatus

PLATE 96

Nematoda (PHASMID NEMATODES, Cont.)

SUPERFAMILY	SIZE and SHAPE	MOUTH and OESOPHAGUS	TAIL IN MALE	REPRODUCTION	GENUS	SPECIES
OXYUROIDEA	Small, ♀ pin shaped	No true capsule 3 lips Distinct posterior bulb in oesophagus	Bursa poorly developed or absent	Oviparous	ENTEROBIUS	VERMICULARIS
ASCAROIDEA	Large, stout	No buccal capsule 3 lips	No bursa	Oviparous	ASCARIS Toxocara Toxocara	LUMBRICOIDES canis cati
SPIRUROIDEA	Filiform to robust	No capsule Various lips	No bursa Various papillae	Oviparous	Gongylonema Gnathostoma Physaloptera Thelazia	pulchrum spinigerum caucasica callipaeda
FILARIOIDEA	Filiform	Rudimentary capsule No lips	Various papillae	Larviparous	WUCHERERIA BRUGIA Brugia Brugia ONCHOCERCA LOA Acanthochielonema Dipetalonema Mansonella Dirofilaria	BANCROFTI MALAYI pahangi patei VOLVULUS LOA perstans streptocerca ozzardi spp.
DRACUNCULOIDEA	Long, cord-like	Mouth simple Oesophagus and intestine rudimentary		Larviparous	DRACUNCULUS	MEDINENSIS

Aphasmid Nematodes

PLATE 97

TRICHINELLA SPIRALIS

Morphology

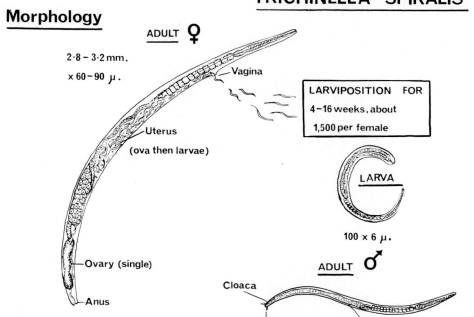

ADULT ♀

2·8 – 3·2 mm.
× 60 – 90 μ.

Vagina

Uterus
(ova then larvae)

LARVIPOSITION FOR
4 – 16 weeks, about
1,500 per female

LARVA

100 × 6 μ.

ADULT ♂

Cloaca

2 conspicuous
conical papillae

Testes

Ovary (single)

Anus

ACTUAL SIZE

Detail anteriorly

Simple mouth
Nerve ring
Oesophagus
Pseudo-bulb

Body cells

Midgut

LIFE CYCLE, PATHOLOGY, OCCURRENCE :– See Plates 7–8

TRICHURIS TRICHIURA

(The Whip worm)

Morphology

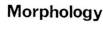

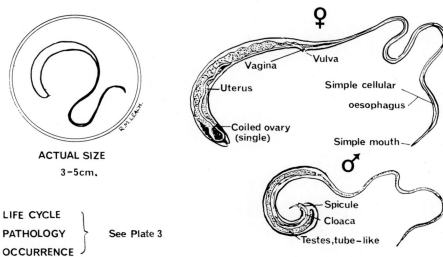

♀

Vulva

Vagina

Uterus

Coiled ovary
(single)

Simple cellular
oesophagus

Simple mouth

♂

Spicule
Cloaca
Testes, tube–like

ACTUAL SIZE
3–5cm.

LIFE CYCLE
PATHOLOGY } See Plate 3
OCCURRENCE

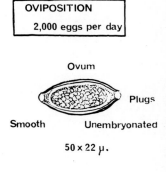

OVIPOSITION
2,000 eggs per day

Ovum

Plugs

Smooth   Unembryonated

50 × 22 μ.

Capillaria hepatica

(The capillary liver worm)

Life cycle

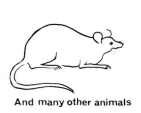

And many other animals

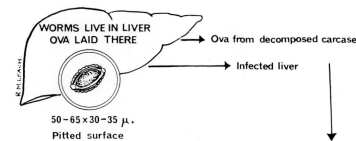

WORMS LIVE IN LIVER
OVA LAID THERE

Ova from decomposed carcase

Infected liver

50 – 65 × 30 – 35 μ.
Pitted surface

New host

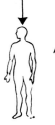

A few true and spurious
infections reported in man

Acute or subacute
hepatitis

Occurrence

Widespread in many animals

PLATE 98

Aphasmid Nematodes (Cont.)

Mermithid worms (including Cabbage snakes)

Morphology

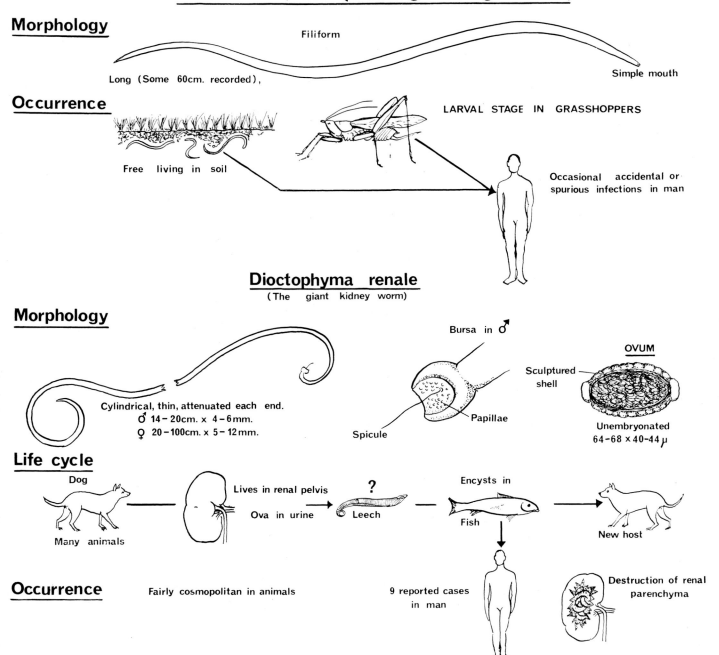

Filiform

Long (Some 60cm. recorded),

Simple mouth

Occurrence

LARVAL STAGE IN GRASSHOPPERS

Free living in soil

Occasional accidental or spurious infections in man

Dioctophyma renale
(The giant kidney worm)

Morphology

Bursa in ♂

OVUM

Sculptured shell

Cylindrical, thin, attenuated each end.
♂ 14 – 20cm. x 4 – 6mm.
♀ 20 – 100cm. x 5 – 12mm.

Spicule

Papillae

Unembryonated
64-68 × 40-44 μ

Life cycle

Dog

Many animals

Lives in renal pelvis

Ova in urine

? Leech

Encysts in

Fish

New host

9 reported cases in man

Destruction of renal parenchyma

Occurrence

Fairly cosmopolitan in animals

Phasmid Nematodes

Strongyloides stercoralis

Morphology

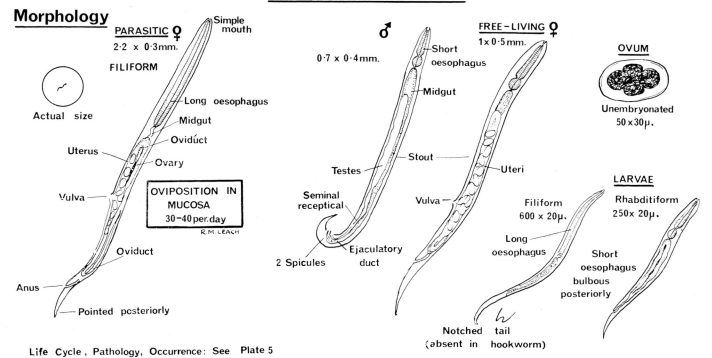

PARASITIC ♀
2·2 x 0·3mm.

FILIFORM

Simple mouth

Actual size

Long oesophagus

Midgut

Oviduct

Uterus

Ovary

Vulva

OVIPOSITION IN MUCOSA
30–40 per. day

R.M. LEACH

Oviduct

Anus

Pointed posteriorly

♂
0·7 x 0·4mm.

Short oesophagus

Midgut

Stout

Testes

Seminal receptical

2 Spicules

Ejaculatory duct

FREE – LIVING ♀
1 x 0·5mm.

Uteri

Vulva

Filiform
600 x 20μ.

Long oesophagus

Notched tail
(absent in hookworm)

OVUM

Unembryonated
50 x 30μ.

LARVAE

Rhabditiform
250 x 20μ.

Short oesophagus bulbous posteriorly

Life Cycle, Pathology, Occurrence: See Plate 5

PLATE 99

Phasmid Nematodes (Cont.)

HOOKWORMS

General morphology

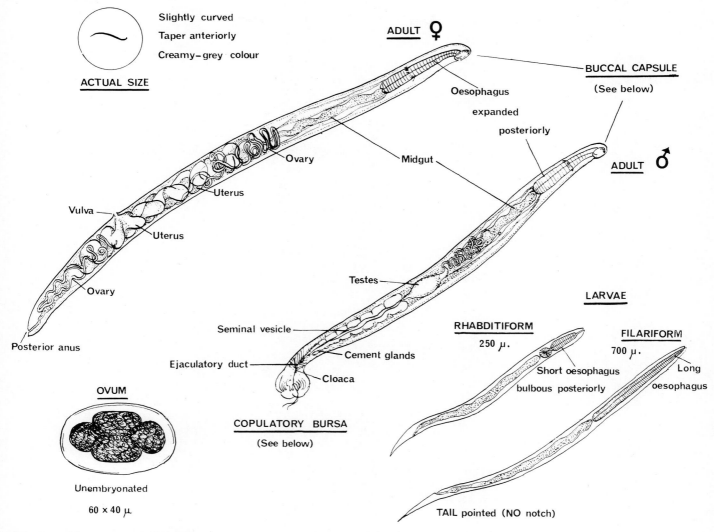

ACTUAL SIZE

Slightly curved
Taper anteriorly
Creamy-grey colour

ADULT ♀

BUCCAL CAPSULE
(See below)

Oesophagus
expanded
posteriorly

Ovary

Midgut

ADULT ♂

Uterus

Vulva

Uterus

Ovary

Posterior anus

Testes

Seminal vesicle

Ejaculatory duct

Cement glands

Cloaca

COPULATORY BURSA
(See below)

LARVAE

RHABDITIFORM
250 μ.

FILARIFORM
700 μ.

Short oesophagus
bulbous posteriorly

Long
oesophagus

OVUM

Unembryonated

60 x 40 μ

TAIL pointed (NO notch)

Particular morphology

Size in mm,	Ancylostoma duodenale	A.braziliense	A. caninum	Necator americanus
♂	8–11 x 0·45.	7·5–8·5 x 0·35.	10 x 0·4.	7–9 x 0·3.
♀	10–13 x 0·6.	9–10·5 x 0·375.	14 x 0·6.	9–11 x 0·4.

BUCCAL CAPSULE

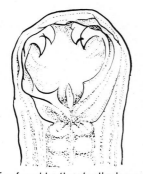 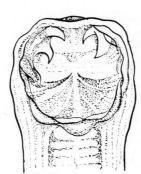 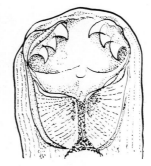 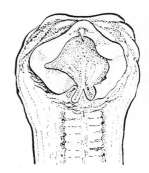

Two fused teeth, outer the larger

2 inconspicuous teeth

Pair of small median teeth

Pair of large outer teeth

Three pairs of teeth

Cutting plates

Dorsal teeth

COPULATORY BURSA

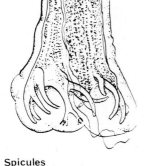 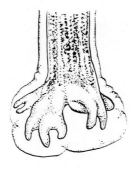 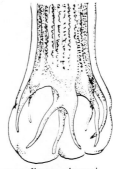 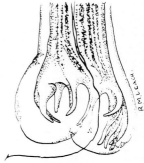

Spicules

Dorsal ray. Shallow cleft

Tips tridigitate

As broad as long

Rays stunted

Large, flame-shaped

Rays long and slender

Spicules fused and barbed

Dorsal ray. Deep cleft.

Tips bifid

PLATE 100

Phasmid Nematodes (HOOKWORMS, Cont.)

ANCYLOSTOMA DUODENALE

Morphology – PLATE 99

LIFE CYCLE ⎫
PATHOLOGY ⎬ SEE PLATE 6
OCCURRENCE ⎭

```
OVIPOSITION
25,000 — 30,000 per. day
```

Ancylostoma braziliense

Animal Strains

OCCURRENCE

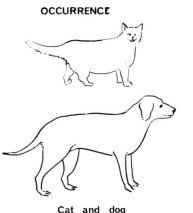

Cat and dog

Life cycle similar to
A. duodenale

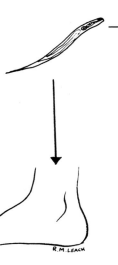

New hosts

SEE PLATE 109

CUTANEOUS LARVA MIGRANS
IF LARVAE OF ANIMAL SPECIES
TRY TO INFECT MAN.
(CREEPING ERUPTION)

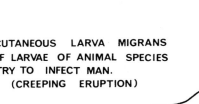

R.M.LEACH

Human Strains

Differ only morphologically from A. duodenale

Ancylostoma caninum

OCCURRENCE

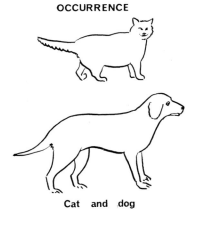

Cat and dog

Life cycle similar to
A. duodenale

CUTANEOUS LARVA MIGRANS.
IF LARVAE ATTEMPT TO INFECT
MAN.

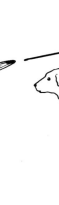

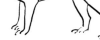

New hosts

SEE PLATE 109

NECATOR AMERICANUS

Morphology – SEE PLATE 99

LIFE CYCLE ⎫
PATHOLOGY ⎬ SEE PLATE 6
OCCURRENCE ⎭

```
OVIPOSITION
10,000 per. day
```

PLATE 101

Phasmid Nematodes (Cont.)

Ternidens deminutus

Morphology

Resemble hookworms but:

♂ Size in mm.
9·5 x 0·56.
♀ 12 – 16 x 0·65.

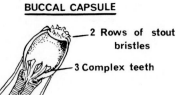

BUCCAL CAPSULE
— 2 Rows of stout bristles
— 3 Complex teeth

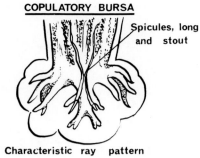

COPULATORY BURSA
Spicules, long and stout
Characteristic ray pattern

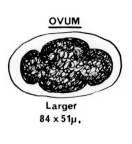

OVUM
Larger
84 x 51μ.

Occurrence

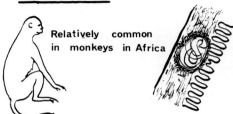 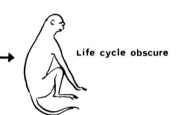

Relatively common in monkeys in Africa

Worms produce cystic nodules in mucosa of large bowel →

Life cycle obscure →

Man occasionally infected

Oesophagostomum apiostomum

Morphology

Like hookworm but

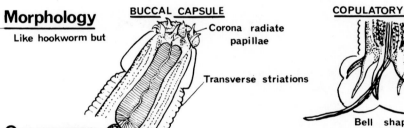

BUCCAL CAPSULE
— Corona radiate papillae
— Transverse striations

COPULATORY BURSA
Bell shaped
Characteristic ray pattern

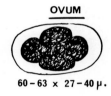

OVUM
60 – 63 x 27 – 40 μ.

Occurrence

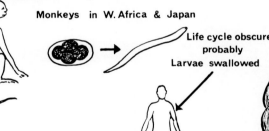

Monkeys in W. Africa & Japan →

Life cycle obscure probably
Larvae swallowed

Man occasionally infected

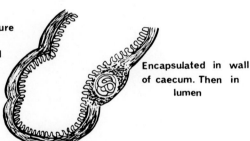

Encapsulated in wall of caecum. Then in lumen

Dysenteric syndrome when nodules break into lumen. Peritonitis if rupture into peritoeum

Syngamus laryngeus

Morphology

Like hookworms but:

♂ and ♀ permanently joined

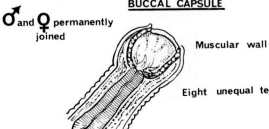

BUCCAL CAPSULE
Muscular wall
Eight unequal teeth

COPULATORY BURSA
Small spicules
Characteristic ray pattern

OVUM
Unembryonated
Sculptured

Occurrence

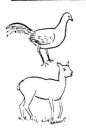

Wide spread in birds and mammals

Ova in sputum →

Life cycle obscure, possibly via earthworms →

New host

Live in trachea

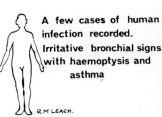

A few cases of human infection recorded. Irritative bronchial signs with haemoptysis and asthma

R.M LEACH.

Trichostrongylus spp.

Morphology

Small, slender. No distinct buccal capsule.

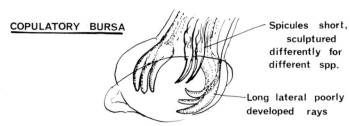

COPULATORY BURSA

Spicules short, sculptured differently for different spp.

Long lateral poorly developed rays

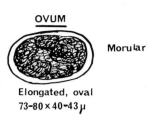

OVUM

Morular

Elongated, oval
73-80 × 40-43 μ

Occurrence

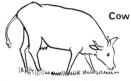

Cow

Frequent in herbivores throughout the world

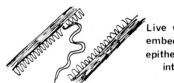

Live with heads embedded in epithelium small intestine

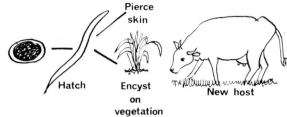

Pierce skin

Hatch

Encyst on vegetation

New host

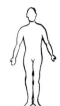

Frequent in man in Asia including U.S.S.R

Traumatic damage to mucosa
May suck blood

Haemonchus contortus
(THE SHEEP WIRE-WORM)

Morphology

Size in mm.

♂ 10-20 × 0·4.

♀ 18-30 × 0·5.

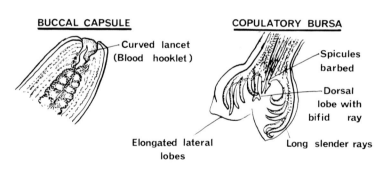

BUCCAL CAPSULE

Curved lancet (Blood hooklet)

Elongated lateral lobes

COPULATORY BURSA

Spicules barbed

Dorsal lobe with bifid ray

Long slender rays

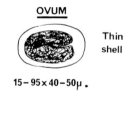

OVUM

Thin shell

15-95 × 40-50 μ.

Occurrence

Sheep

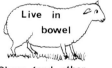

Live in bowel

Sheep (and other herbivores) through-out the world

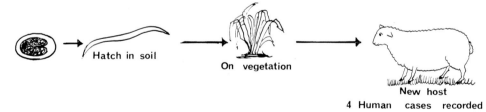

Hatch in soil

On vegetation

New host

4 Human cases recorded

Metastrongylus elongatus
(THE PORCINE LUNG WORM)

Morphology

Size in mm.

♂ 12-25 × 1·6-2·2.

♀ 20-58 × 4-4·5.

MOUTH

No buccal capsule

Pair of lateral tri-lobed lips

COPULATORY BURSA

Bilobed

Ray swollen at tip

OVUM

Thick shell

Embryonated
51-54 × 33-36 μ.

Occurrence

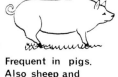

Frequent in pigs. Also sheep and cattle

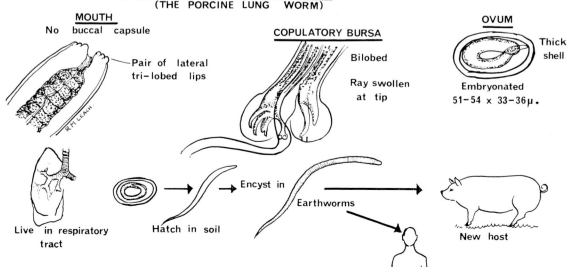

Live in respiratory tract

Hatch in soil

Encyst in

Earthworms

New host

3 Human cases reported

ENTEROBIUS VERMICULARIS
(THE PIN WORM)

Morphology

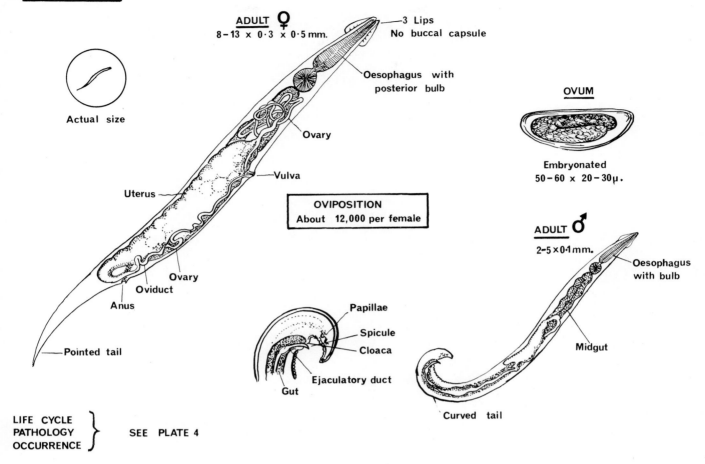

ADULT ♀
8 – 13 x 0·3 x 0·5 mm.

3 Lips
No buccal capsule

Actual size

Oesophagus with posterior bulb

OVUM

Ovary

Embryonated
50 – 60 x 20 – 30μ.

Uterus

Vulva

OVIPOSITION
About 12,000 per female

ADULT ♂
2-5 x 0·1 mm.

Ovary

Oviduct

Oesophagus with bulb

Anus

Papillae
Spicule
Cloaca

Pointed tail

Midgut

Gut

Ejaculatory duct

Curved tail

LIFE CYCLE
PATHOLOGY
OCCURRENCE } SEE PLATE 4

ASCARIS LUMBRICOIDES
(THE ROUND WORM OF THE INTESTINE)

Morphology

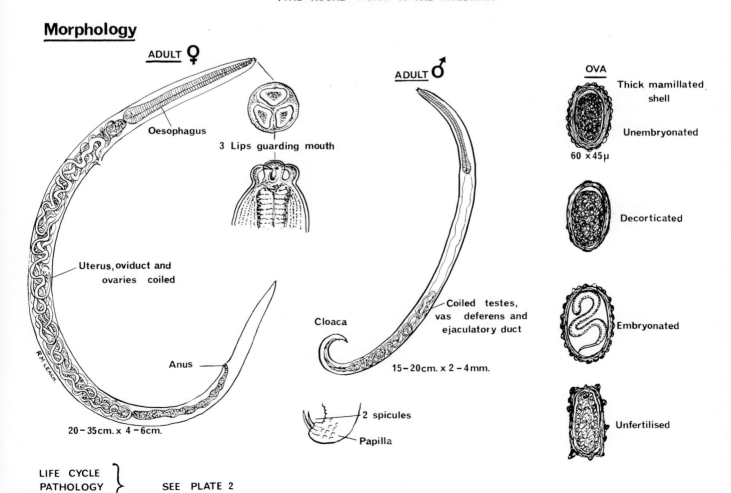

ADULT ♀

ADULT ♂

OVA

Oesophagus

Thick mamillated shell

3 Lips guarding mouth

Unembryonated

60 x 45μ

Uterus, oviduct and ovaries coiled

Decorticated

Coiled testes, vas deferens and ejaculatory duct

Cloaca

Embryonated

Anus

15 – 20cm. x 2 – 4 mm.

20 – 35 cm. x 4 – 6 cm.

2 spicules

Unfertilised

Papilla

LIFE CYCLE
PATHOLOGY
OCCURRENCE } SEE PLATE 2

PLATE 104

Phasmid Nematodes (Cont)

Toxocara canis
(THE DOG ROUND WORM)

Morphology

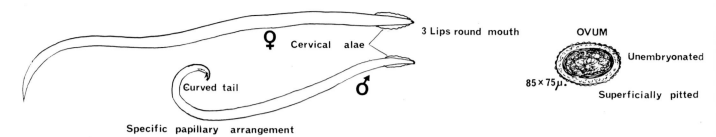

♀ Cervical alae — 3 Lips round mouth
Curved tail
♂
Specific papillary arrangement

OVUM
Unembryonated
85 × 75 µ.
Superficially pitted

Life cycle

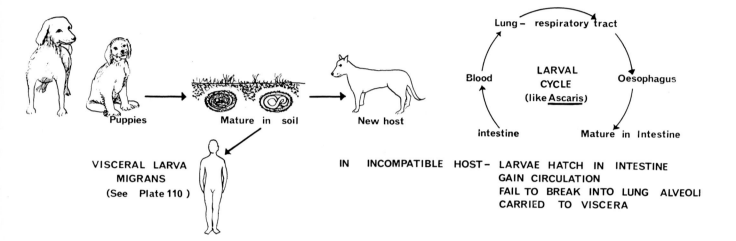

Puppies — Mature in soil — New host

VISCERAL LARVA MIGRANS
(See Plate 110)

Lung – respiratory tract
Blood — LARVAL CYCLE (like *Ascaris*) — Oesophagus
intestine — Mature in Intestine

IN INCOMPATIBLE HOST – LARVAE HATCH IN INTESTINE
GAIN CIRCULATION
FAIL TO BREAK INTO LUNG ALVEOLI
CARRIED TO VISCERA

Toxocara cati
(THE CAT ROUND WORM)

Morphology

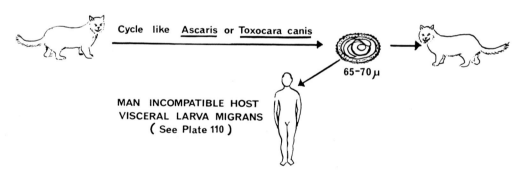

Cycle like *Ascaris* or *Toxocara canis*
65-70 µ

MAN INCOMPATIBLE HOST
VISCERAL LARVA MIGRANS
(See Plate 110)

Gongylonema pulchrum
(THE SCUTATE THREADWORM)

Morphology

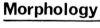

Long and thin
♀ 14.5 × 0.2 – 0.5 cm.
♂ 6.2 × 0.15 – 0.3 cm.

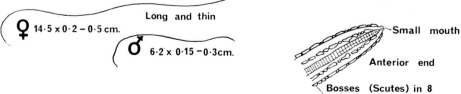

Small mouth
Anterior end
Bosses (Scutes) in 8 longitudinal series

OVUM
Embryonated
Thick shell
50 – 70 × 25 – 37 µ.

Life cycle and occurrence

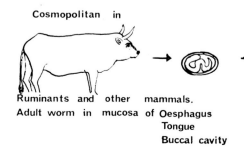

Cosmopolitan in

Ruminants and other mammals.
Adult worm in mucosa of Oesphagus
Tongue
Buccal cavity

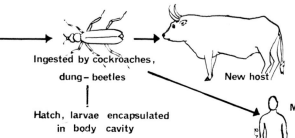

Ingested by cockroaches, dung – beetles

Hatch, larvae encapsulated in body cavity

New host

Larvae liberated in duodenum, migrate to buccal cavity. Move in tunnel in mucosa

Man occasionally infected (18 cases recorded)

GONGYLONEMIASIS

PLATE 105

Phasmid Nematodes (Cont)

Gnathostoma spinigerum

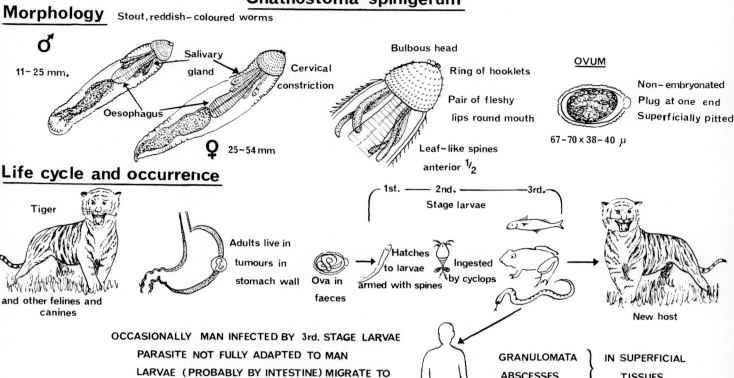

Morphology Stout, reddish-coloured worms

♂ 11-25 mm.

Salivary gland
Oesophagus
Cervical constriction

♀ 25-54 mm

Bulbous head
Ring of hooklets
Pair of fleshy lips round mouth
Leaf-like spines anterior ½

OVUM
Non-embryonated
Plug at one end
Superficially pitted
67-70 × 38-40 μ

Life cycle and occurrence

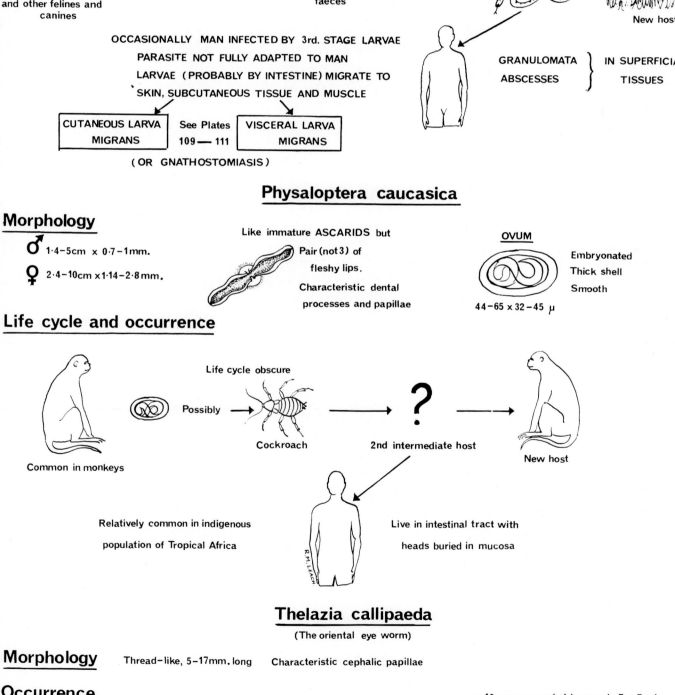

Tiger
and other felines and canines

Adults live in tumours in stomach wall

Ova in faeces

Hatches to larvae armed with spines

Ingested by cyclops

1st. — 2nd. — 3rd.
Stage larvae

New host

OCCASIONALLY MAN INFECTED BY 3rd. STAGE LARVAE
PARASITE NOT FULLY ADAPTED TO MAN
LARVAE (PROBABLY BY INTESTINE) MIGRATE TO
SKIN, SUBCUTANEOUS TISSUE AND MUSCLE

GRANULOMATA
ABSCESSES } IN SUPERFICIAL TISSUES

| CUTANEOUS LARVA MIGRANS | See Plates 109 — 111 | VISCERAL LARVA MIGRANS |

(OR GNATHOSTOMIASIS)

Physaloptera caucasica

Morphology

♂ 1·4-5cm × 0·7-1mm.
♀ 2·4-10cm × 1·14-2·8mm.

Like immature ASCARIDS but
Pair (not 3) of fleshy lips.
Characteristic dental processes and papillae

OVUM
Embryonated
Thick shell
Smooth
44-65 × 32-45 μ

Life cycle and occurrence

Common in monkeys

Life cycle obscure
Possibly
Cockroach
?
2nd intermediate host
New host

Relatively common in indigenous population of Tropical Africa

Live in intestinal tract with heads buried in mucosa

Thelazia callipaeda
(The oriental eye worm)

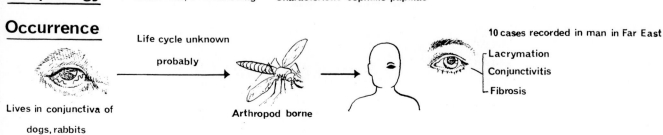

Morphology Thread-like, 5-17mm. long Characteristic cephalic papillae

Occurrence

Lives in conjunctiva of dogs, rabbits

Life cycle unknown probably
Arthropod borne

10 cases recorded in man in Far East
Lacrymation
Conjunctivitis
Fibrosis

PLATE 106

Phasmid Nematodes (Cont.)

The Filarial Worms

Morphology

ADULTS

LARVAL FORMS

Microfilaria sheathed
Note: Egg shell elongated round embryo

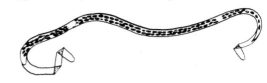

Microfilaria unsheathed   Egg shell lost

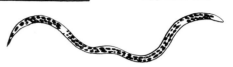

Columns of nuclei (developing organs) used in identification

Wuchereria bancrofti

♂ Minute, creamy white, thread-like
4 x 1·0 cm.

Two unequal spicules

♀

8·10 x 0·3 cm.

Mouth unarmed
No buccal capule
2 rows of sessile papillae

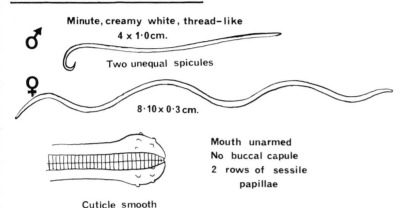

Cuticle smooth

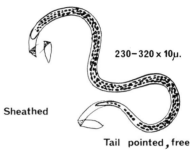

230–320 x 10μ.

Sheathed

Tail pointed, free from nuclei

Brugia malayi

In general like **W. bancrofti**

2 rows minute papillae round mouth

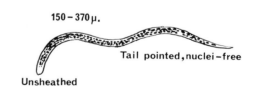

170–260 x 5–6μ.

Sheathed

Two discrete nuclei in tip of tail

Onchocerca volvulus

♂ 2–4 cm. x 130–210μ.
♀ 33–50 cm. x 270–400μ.

Papillae round mouth

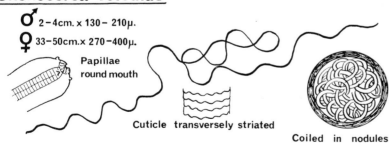

Cuticle transversely striated

Coiled in nodules

150–370μ.

Tail pointed, nuclei–free

Unsheathed

Loa loa

♂ 3–3·4 cm. x 0·4 mm.   Thread like
♀ 5–7 cm. x 0·5 mm.

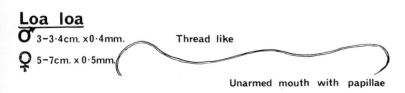

Unarmed mouth with papillae

Nuclei to tip of tail

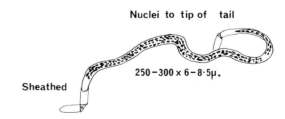

250–300 x 6–8·5μ.

Sheathed

Acanthochielonema (Dipetalonema) perstans

♂ 4·5 cm. x 60μ.
♀ 7·8 cm. x 120μ.

Bifurcated posteriorly   Papillae anteriorly

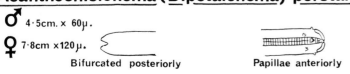

Unsheathed   200 x 4·5μ.   Tail blunt
Nuclei to tip

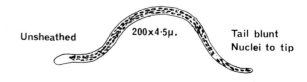

Tail blunt, curved
Nuclei almost to tip

Unsheathed

Dipetalonema streptocerca

Little studied

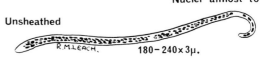

R.M.LEACH.   180–240 x 3μ.

PLATE 107

Phasmid Nematodes (Filarial Worms, Cont.)

Morphology of filarial worms, continued

ADULTS   LARVAL FORMS

Mansonella ozzardi

♂ not studied

♀ 6-8 cm. by 0·25 mm.

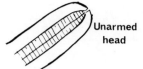

Unsheathed   Tip of tail free from nuclei

Unarmed head

Cuticle smooth

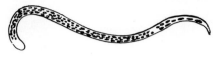

175-240 by 4·5 μ.

Pair of fleshy flaps posteriorly

Life cycle, Pathology and Occurrence of Filarial Worms

WUCHERERIA BANCROFTI   see Plate 9

BRUGIA MALAYI   see Plate 10

    B. pahangi   }   Parasites of cat and dog families

    B. patei   Microfilaria may cause Tropical Eosinophilia, see Plates 110–111

LOA LOA   see   Plate 11

ONCHOCERCA VOLVULUS   see   Plate 12

DIPETALONEMA (ACANTHOCHEILONEMA) PERSTANS

    Live in body cavities (especially peritoneal) of Man and Monkeys

    Spread by CULICOIDES

    Microfilaria in blood (not strictly periodic)

    Widespread in Tropical Africa and America

    No definite pathogenicity

DIPETALONEMA STREPTOCERCA

    Life cycle obscure

    Widespread in MAN in Gold Coast, described elsewhere in Africa, possibly India.

    Microfilaria in blood

    No definite pathogenicity

MANSONELLA OZZARDI

    Live in body cavities of Man

    Microfilaria in blood

    Found in Tropical America

    No definite pathogenicity

PLATE 108

Phasmid Nematodes (Filarial worms, Cont.)

Dirofilaria Spp.

Described in various situations, life cycle obscure

D. conjuntivae   Lives encysted in subcutaneous tissue

D. immitis   A dog parasite, lives in cardiac chamber.

Usual source of antigen (group-specific) for intradermal and complement fixation tests for filarial infections in man

Phasmid Nematodes (Cont.)

DRACUNCULUS MEDINENSIS
(The guinea worm)

Morphology

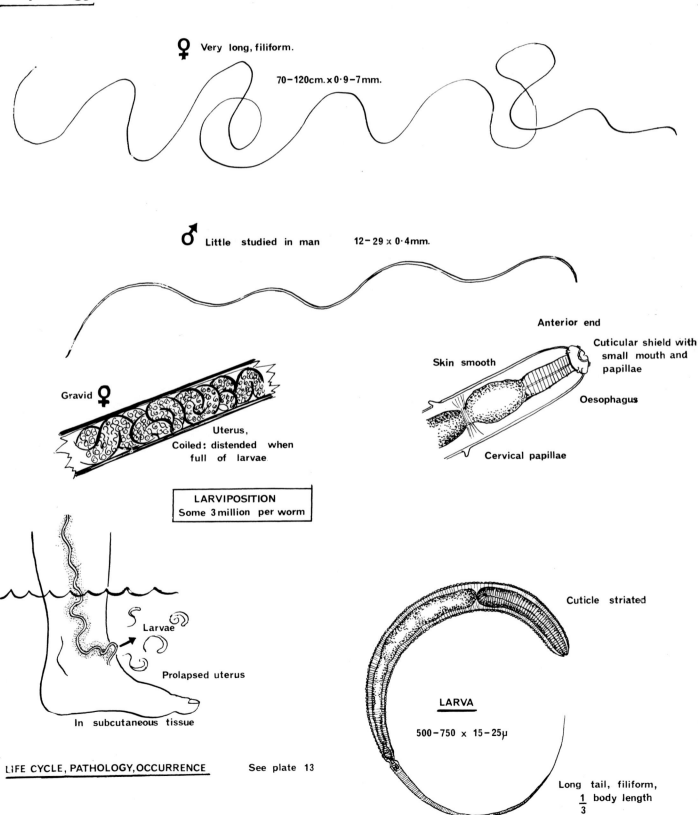

♀ Very long, filiform.

70-120cm. x 0·9-7mm.

♂ Little studied in man   12-29 x 0·4mm.

Gravid ♀

Uterus,
Coiled: distended when full of larvae

Anterior end

Skin smooth

Cuticular shield with small mouth and papillae

Oesophagus

Cervical papillae

LARVIPOSITION
Some 3 million per worm

Larvae

Prolapsed uterus

In subcutaneous tissue

Cuticle striated

LARVA

500-750 x 15-25µ

Long tail, filiform, $\frac{1}{3}$ body length

LIFE CYCLE, PATHOLOGY, OCCURRENCE   See plate 13

PLATE 109

Phasmid Nematodes (Cont)

LARVA MIGRANS

Larvae of certain nematodes in aberrant sites ⟨ cutaneous
visceral

CUTANEOUS LARVA MIGRANS (CREEPING ERUPTION)

1. Typically due to Non-Human Hookworm Larvae

NORMAL CYCLE

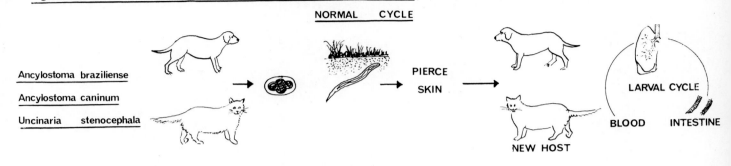

Ancylostoma braziliense

Ancylostoma caninum

Uncinaria stenocephala

PIERCE SKIN

NEW HOST

LARVAL CYCLE

BLOOD   INTESTINE

IF ATTEMPT TO INVADE MAN

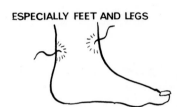

ESPECIALLY FEET AND LEGS

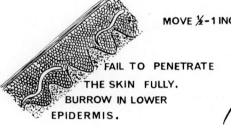

MOVE ½-1 INCH PER DAY

FAIL TO PENETRATE THE SKIN FULLY. BURROW IN LOWER EPIDERMIS.

INTENSELY ITCHY
SECONDARY INFECTION
LASTS MONTHS

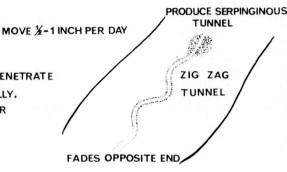

PRODUCE SERPINGINOUS TUNNEL

ZIG ZAG TUNNEL

FADES OPPOSITE END

2. Sometimes due to Gnathostoma spinigerum

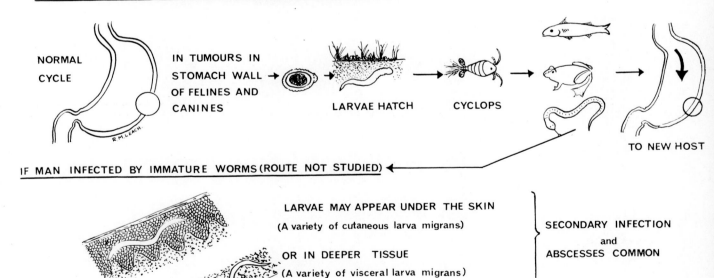

NORMAL CYCLE

IN TUMOURS IN STOMACH WALL OF FELINES AND CANINES

LARVAE HATCH

CYCLOPS

TO NEW HOST

IF MAN INFECTED BY IMMATURE WORMS (ROUTE NOT STUDIED)

LARVAE MAY APPEAR UNDER THE SKIN
(A variety of cutaneous larva migrans)

OR IN DEEPER TISSUE
(A variety of visceral larva migrans)

⟩ SECONDARY INFECTION and ABSCESSES COMMON

3. Sometimes due to Non-Helminth Agents

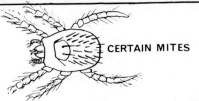

CERTAIN MITES

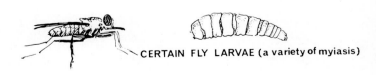

CERTAIN FLY LARVAE (a variety of myiasis)

LABORATORY DIAGNOSIS OF CUTANEOUS LARVA MIGRANS

Surgically removed larvae

Recognition under skin (cleared with mineral oil)

PLATE 110

Nematodes (Larva migrans, Cont.)

VISCERAL LARVA MIGRANS

<u>Definition</u> INFECTION BY **1 Larvae of non-human nematodes attempting to invade man Fail to complete normal life cycle**

2 Larvae of human nematodes getting lost in ectopic sites

<u>AETIOLOGY</u> SUGGESTED CLASSIFICATION **1. Due to non-human nematodes**

A. CLASSICAL TYPE: INGESTION OF EMBRYONATED OVA OF DOG & CAT ROUND WORMS

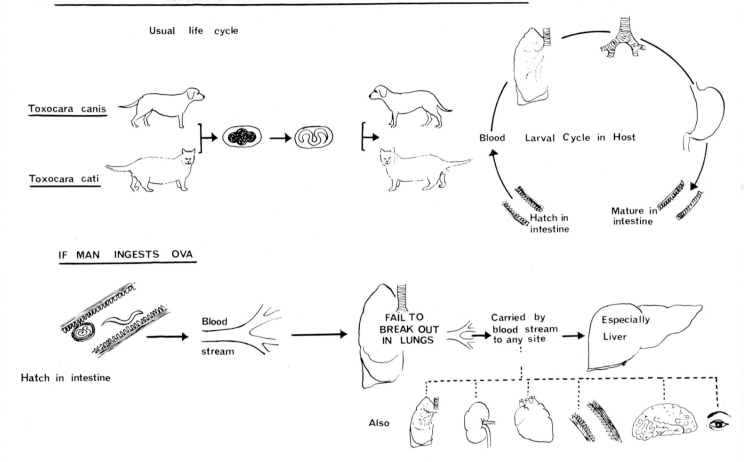

Usual life cycle

Toxocara canis

Toxocara cati

Blood Larval Cycle in Host

Hatch in intestine

Mature in intestine

IF MAN INGESTS OVA

Hatch in intestine

Blood stream

FAIL TO BREAK OUT IN LUNGS

Carried by blood stream to any site

Especially Liver

Also

B. NON-HUMAN HOOKWORMS

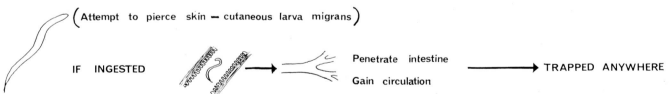

(Attempt to pierce skin — cutaneous larva migrans)

IF INGESTED

Penetrate intestine

Gain circulation → TRAPPED ANYWHERE

C. GNATHOSTOMA SPINIGERUM (See plate 105)

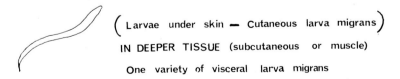

(Larvae under skin — Cutaneous larva migrans)

IN DEEPER TISSUE (subcutaneous or muscle)

One variety of visceral larva migrans

D. NON-HUMAN FILARIAL Spp

Microfilaria are possible cause of Tropical Eosinophilia

Serum gives + C.F.T. for filaria

Spp. incriminated <u>Dirofilaria immitis</u> (The dog filaria)

<u>Brugia pahangi</u>
<u>Brugia patei</u> } parasites of dogs & cats

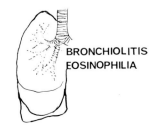

BRONCHIOLITIS EOSINOPHILIA

Aetiology, continued   ## 2. Due to human nematodes

A. LARVAE OF <u>ASCARIS LUMBRICOIDES</u> (IN HEAVY INFECTIONS)

<u>STRONGYLOIDES STERCORALIS</u> (IN AUTO—AND HYPER-INFECTIONS)

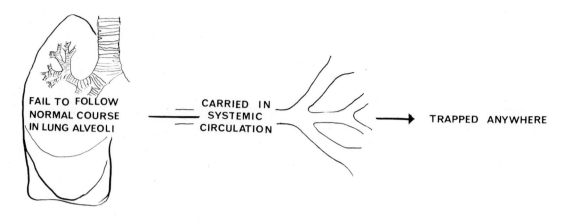

FAIL TO FOLLOW NORMAL COURSE IN LUNG ALVEOLI — CARRIED IN SYSTEMIC CIRCULATION → TRAPPED ANYWHERE

B. MICROFILARIA OF <u>BRUGIA MALAYI</u> CAN CAUSE A SYNDROME LIKE TROPICAL EOSINOPHILIA.

PATHOLOGY

1. Larva trapped in tissue

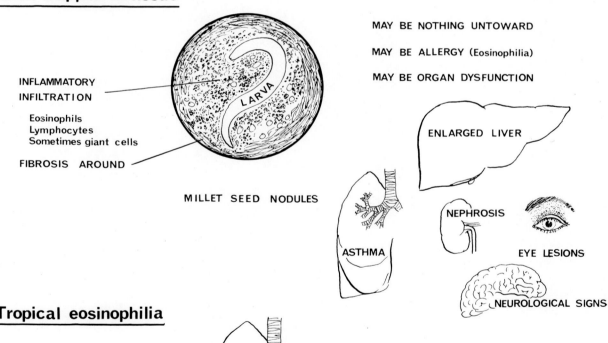

INFLAMMATORY INFILTRATION

Eosinophils
Lymphocytes
Sometimes giant cells

FIBROSIS AROUND

LARVA

MILLET SEED NODULES

MAY BE NOTHING UNTOWARD

MAY BE ALLERGY (Eosinophilia)

MAY BE ORGAN DYSFUNCTION

ENLARGED LIVER

ASTHMA

NEPHROSIS

EYE LESIONS

NEUROLOGICAL SIGNS

2. Tropical eosinophilia

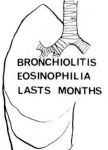

BRONCHIOLITIS
EOSINOPHILIA
LASTS MONTHS

LABORATORY DIAGNOSIS OF VISCERAL LARVA MIGRANS

Histology of biopsy specimens

Serological in some cases (e.g. Complement Fixation Test in Tropical Eosinophilia.)

Intradermal tests in some cases (e.g. <u>Toxocara</u>.)

Miscellaneous Worms

PLATE 112

Phylum   NEMATOPHORA. (Gordiid worms or hair snakes)

Class   GORDIACEA. Elongated, wiry worms 10-50 cm. long. Digestive tract atrophied.

LIFE CYCLE

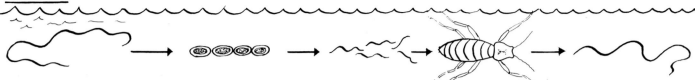

Free living in water   Ova   Larvae hatch   Penetrate intermediate
                                                                            host.   Develop into
                                                                            adolescent worms

                                                                            Escape from insect
                                                                            Mature in water

Man may ingest   Free living adults
                  Adolescents in insects

                  Many species cause spurious infections in man

                                                                            In intestine
                                                                            In urinary tract occasionally

                  A single   case of   tissue   invasion (the orbit) reported

---

Phylum ACANTHOCEPHALA   Thorny headed   worms

MORPHOLOGY   Possess proboscis armed with spines

♂ 5-10 cm, ♀ 20-65 cm. in length

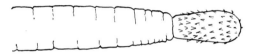

LIFE CYCLE

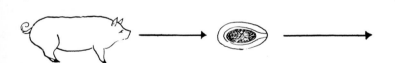

Adults in intestines   Ova in   Arthopod   Insect eaten
of vertebrates   faeces   intermediate host   by new host

Species

Macrocanthorhynchus
hirudinaceus

OVUM
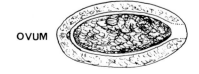

3 envelopes

80 - 100 by 40-50 μ.

Cosmopolitan in pigs

A few spurious infections
reported in man

Moniliformis
moniliformis

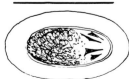

3 envelopes
Spinose embryo
85 - 118 by 40 - 52 μ.

Found in rats

Solitary human infections reported in
man in Italy, Sudan and British Honduras

Recapitulation
Ova of the less common or less important worms

PLATE 113

CESTODA

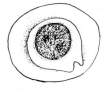
Bertiella studeri

Dipylidium caninum

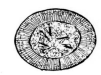
Multiceps multiceps

TREMATODA

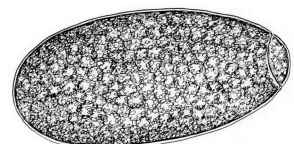
Fasciola gigantica

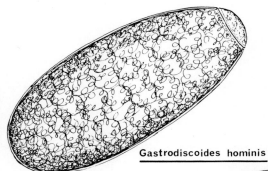
Gastrodiscoides hominis

Dicrocoelium denditricum

Opisthorchis felineus

Heterophyes heterophyes

Metagonimus yokagawai

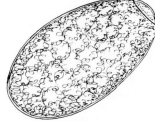
Echinostoma ilocanum

0   50   100 μ

NEMATODA

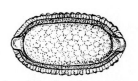
Capillaria hepatica

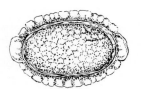
Dioctophyma renale

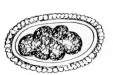
Syngamus laryngeus

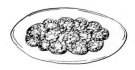
Trichostrongylus spp.

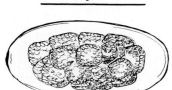
Haemonchus contortus

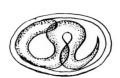
Metastrongylus elongatus

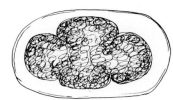
Ternidens deminutus

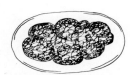
Oesophagostomum apiostomomum
(like hookworm)

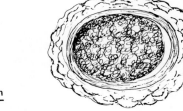
Toxocara spp.
(ova in dogs & cats)

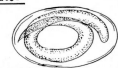
Physaloptera caucasica

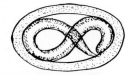
Gongylonema pulchrum

MISCELLANEOUS WORMS

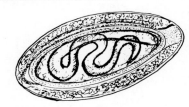
Macracanthorhynchus hirudinaceus

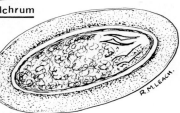
Moniliformis moniliformis

PATHOGENESIS and PATHOLOGY of WORM INFECTIONS

FACTORS

Generally DO NOT MULTIPLY IN MAN	Generally NOT IN INTIMATE TISSUE CONTACT
Repeated or massive attacks before effects are apparent	Immunity response poor

OFFENCE and DEFENCE

METABOLITES (Alive) DECOMPOSITION PRODUCTS (Dead)	SIZE MECHANICAL PRESSURE & OBSTRUCTIVE EFFECTS	EXCITATION OF LOCAL TISSUE REACTION	ABSORPTION OF NOURISHMENT

GENERAL EFFECTS   LOCAL TISSUE EFFECTS

---

1. GENERAL EFFECTS

	Clinico – pathological correlation

TOXAEMIA & ALLERGY

<u>ACUTE</u> DURING LARVAL INVASION e.g. Ancylostomiasis

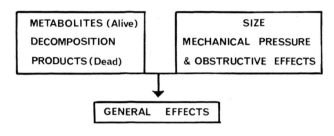

Ascariasis
Trichiniasis

OVA INVASION

Schistosomiasis

CHRONIC ILL DEFINED
    Can occur in any heavy worm infection

Clinico-pathological correlation:
Fever
Eosinophilia

Urticaria
Katayama fever

Irregular fever
Eosinophilia, Urticaria
Nervous disturbance
    especially in children

ANAPHYLAXIS

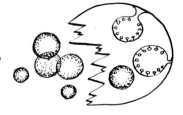

RUPTURE OF CYSTS   e.g. Hydatid disease

Acute anaphylactic shock

MALNUTRITION

eg LARGE TAPEWORM INFECTIONS
    HEAVY NEMATODE INFECTIONS etc.

Loss of weight

Fatigue

ANAEMIA

LOSS OF BLOOD e.g.   Hookworm infections

Anaemia with sequelae

DECREASED GENERAL RESISTANCE

IN ANY PROLONGED, HEAVY INFECTION

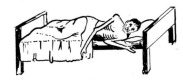

Intercurrent disease

Plate 115

Recapitulation (Cont.)

2. LOCAL EFFECTS   A. GENERAL

Mechanical obstruction

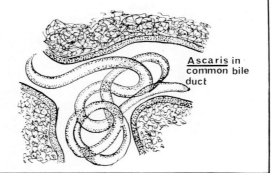

Ascaris in common bile duct

Intestinal obstruction
Appendicitis
Obstructive jaundice
Pancreatitis

Pressure effects

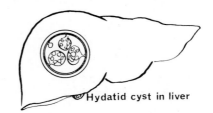

Hydatid cyst in liver

Destruction of parenchyma
Interference with physiological function

Granulomata
around **adults**
larvae
ova

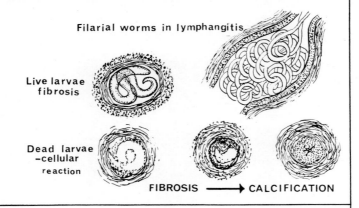

Filarial worms in lymphangitis

Live larvae fibrosis

Dead larvae –cellular reaction

FIBROSIS ⟶ CALCIFICATION

Syndrome referable to site

Space-occupying lesion

include some of above

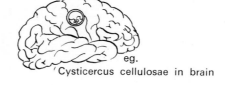

eg.
Cysticercus cellulosae in brain

eg. Focal neurological signs

Damage to epithelium

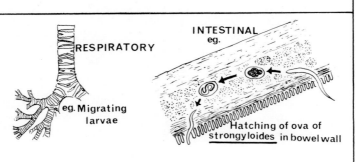

RESPIRATORY

eg. Migrating larvae

INTESTINAL eg.

Hatching of ova of strongyloides in bowel wall

Haemoptysis
Pneumonitis

Diarrhoea or dysentery

Superficial manifestations

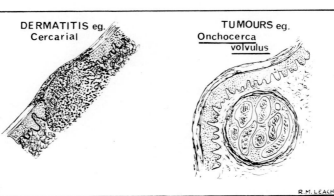

DERMATITIS eg. Cercarial

TUMOURS eg. Onchocerca volvulus

R.M.LEACH

Papular
Macular
Pustular
Vesicular } rashes

Subcutaneous tumours

SECONDARY INFECTION

other COMPLICATIONS & SEQUELAE

PLATE 116

Recapitulation (Cont.)

LOCAL EFFECTS   B. PARTICULAR

The Brain and Spinal Cord

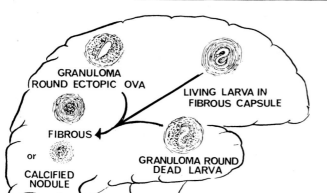

GRANULOMA
ROUND ECTOPIC OVA

LIVING LARVA IN
FIBROUS CAPSULE

FIBROUS

or

CALCIFIED
NODULE

GRANULOMA ROUND
DEAD LARVA

LARVAE

CESTODA CYSTICERCUS CELLULOSAE(T. solium)

COENURUS CEREBRALIS(Multiceps spp)

HYDATID (E. granulosus)

Focal neurological signs
e.g. epilepsy

Space occupying lesions

NEMATODA VISCERAL LARVA MIGRANS

Especially TOXOCARA spp.

Ascaris lumbricoides

Strongyloides stercoralis

ECTOPIC OVA

TREMATODA Schistosoma mansoni and japonicum

Fasciola hepatica

Heterophyes heterophyes

Metagonimus yokogowai

The Eye

ADULTS UNDER CONJUNCTIVA

INVASION OF LARVAE

NEMATODA   ADULTS   LOA LOA

Thelazia callipaeda

Dirofilaria conjunctivae

LARVAE.   Mf. of Onchocerca volvulus

VISCERAL LARVA MIGRANS

eg. Toxocara canis

Irritation
Conjunctivitis
Keratitis
Eye tumour
Blindness

The Mouth and Pharynx

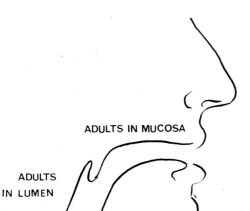

ADULTS IN MUCOSA

ADULTS
IN LUMEN

NEMATODA   Gongylonema pulchrum

Irritation

TREMATODA Spurious infection with

Fasciola hepatica
(Halzoun)

Irritation

Haemoptysis

Local effects of worm infections, continued

The Respiratory Passages and Lungs

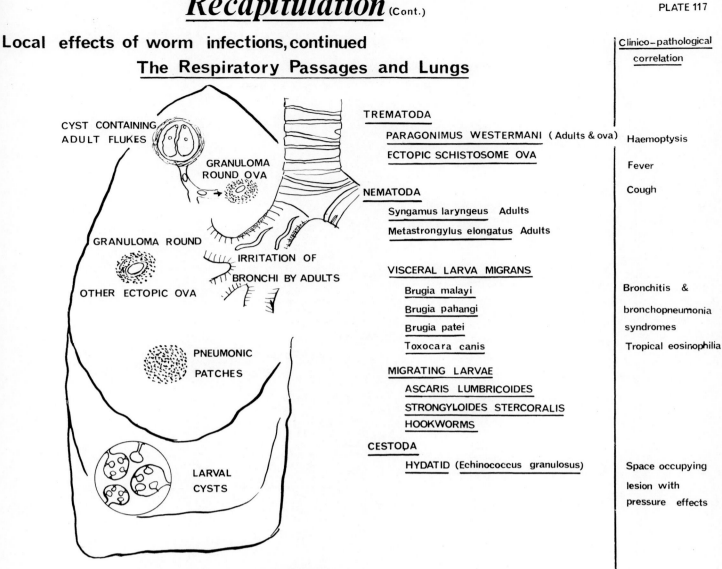

CYST CONTAINING
ADULT FLUKES

GRANULOMA
ROUND OVA

GRANULOMA ROUND

OTHER ECTOPIC OVA

IRRITATION OF
BRONCHI BY ADULTS

PNEUMONIC
PATCHES

LARVAL
CYSTS

TREMATODA

PARAGONIMUS WESTERMANI (Adults & ova)

ECTOPIC SCHISTOSOME OVA

NEMATODA

Syngamus laryngeus   Adults

Metastrongylus elongatus Adults

VISCERAL LARVA MIGRANS

Brugia malayi

Brugia pahangi

Brugia patei

Toxocara canis

MIGRATING LARVAE

ASCARIS LUMBRICOIDES

STRONGYLOIDES STERCORALIS

HOOKWORMS

CESTODA

HYDATID (Echinococcus granulosus)

Haemoptysis

Fever

Cough

Bronchitis &

bronchopneumonia

syndromes

Tropical eosinophilia

Space occupying

lesion with

pressure effects

The Liver and Bile Ducts

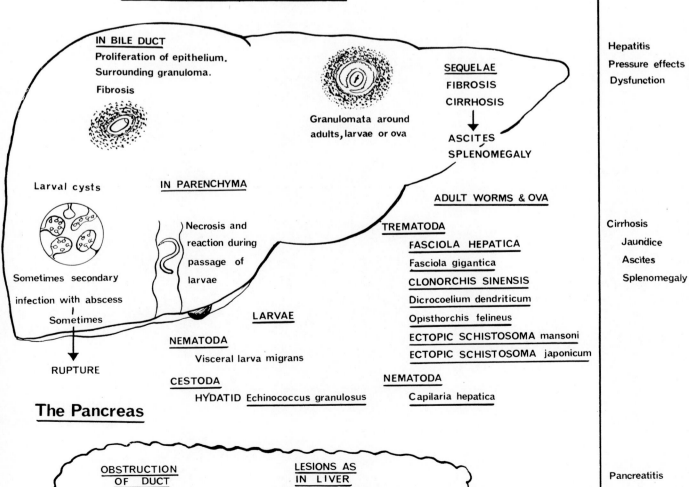

IN BILE DUCT
Proliferation of epithelium.
Surrounding granuloma.
Fibrosis

Granulomata around
adults, larvae or ova

SEQUELAE
FIBROSIS
CIRRHOSIS

ASCITES
SPLENOMEGALY

Larval cysts

IN PARENCHYMA

Necrosis and
reaction during
passage of
larvae

Sometimes secondary

infection with abscess

Sometimes

RUPTURE

LARVAE

NEMATODA
Visceral larva migrans

CESTODA
HYDATID Echinococcus granulosus

ADULT WORMS & OVA

TREMATODA

FASCIOLA HEPATICA

Fasciola gigantica

CLONORCHIS SINENSIS

Dicrocoelium dendriticum

Opisthorchis felineus

ECTOPIC SCHISTOSOMA mansoni

ECTOPIC SCHISTOSOMA japonicum

NEMATODA

Capilaria hepatica

Hepatitis
Pressure effects
Dysfunction

Cirrhosis

Jaundice

Ascites

Splenomegaly

The Pancreas

OBSTRUCTION
OF DUCT

NEMATODA

Ascaris lumbricoides

occasionally

LESIONS AS
IN LIVER

TREMATODA Clonorchis sinensis

Pancreatitis

PLATE 118

Local Effects of Worm Infection, continued

Recapitulation (Cont.)

The Intestinal Tract

NEMATODA

ASCARIS LUMBRICOIDES
TRICHURIS TRICHIURA
ENTEROBIUS VERMICULARIS
Mermithoid worms
Trichostrongylus spp
Physoloptera caucasica
Haemonchus contortus

TREMATODA

FASCIOLOPSIS BUSKI
Watsonius watsoni
Gastrodiscoides hominis
Heterophyes heterophyes
Metagonimus yokagawai
Echinostoma spp.

Clinico–pathologi
correlation

IN VAST MAJOR

ASYMPTOMATIC

SUPERFICIAL MUCOSAL IRRITATION
ABSORPTION OF NUTRIMENT
OCCASIONALLY OBSTRUCTION

CESTODA

TAENIA SOLIUM
TAENIA SAGINATA
DIBOTHRIOCEPHALUS LATUM
Hymenolepis diminuta
Diplogonoporus grandis
Inermicapsifer spp
Bertiella studeri
Dipylidium canium
Railletina spp

Vague adominal
symptoms.
Anorexia, indigest
Colicky pain,
Loss of weight
Diarrhoea
Appendicitis
Obstruction

SUCK BLOOD

NEMATODA

HOOKWORMS ANCYLOSTOMA DUODENALE
Ancylostoma braziliense human strains
NECATOR AMERICANUS
Trichostrongylus spp

Vague abdominal
symptoms
ANAEMIA &
SEQUELAE

May absorb B_{12}
CESTODA
Dibothriocephalus latum

Megaloblastic
anaemia

Perianal irritation
NEMATODA
Enterobius vermicularis

Pruritis ani
and vulvae

ADULTS OR LARVAE
PENETRATE MUCOSA

NEMATODA
STRONGYLOIDES STERCORALIS
Oviposition and hatching in wall

From

COLIC and

DYSENTERY

TRICHINELLA SPIRALIS
Larviposition in wall

To

Slight abdomina

pain

Diarrhoea

Ternidens deminutus &
Oesophagostomum apiostomum
Encapsulated in wall Adult to lumen

GRANULOMATA &
SEQUELAE AROUND OVA

CESTODA

HYMENOLEPIS NANA
Cysticercus in wall
Adult in lumen

GRANULOMA

PAPILLOMA

SECONDARY INFECTION
ULCERS & ABSCESSES

DYSENTERY ear
SEQUELAE wit
Diarrhoea
Obstruction
Ileus
Fistulae
(And extra intes
lesions)

TREMATODA

SCHISTOSOMA MANSONI (Mainly large intestine)
SCHISTOSOMA JAPONICUM (Mainly small intestine)

FIBROSIS

PLATE 119

Recapitulation (Cont.)

Local effects of worm infection, continued

The Urinary Tract

Clinico-pathological
correlation

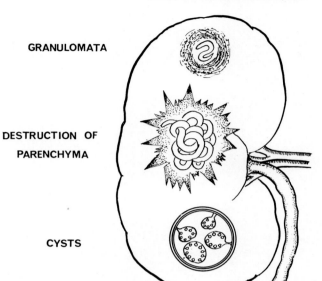

GRANULOMATA

NEMATODA

VISCERAL LARVA MIGRANS

DESTRUCTION OF
PARENCHYMA

Dioctophyma renale

Impaired renal function

CYSTS

CESTODA

HYDATID (Echinococcus granulosus)

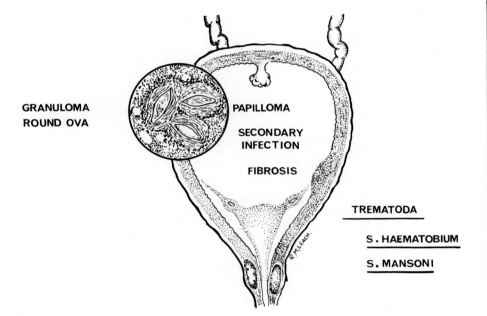

GRANULOMA
ROUND OVA

PAPILLOMA

SECONDARY
INFECTION

FIBROSIS

HAEMATURIA
CYSTITIS

Sequelae including
calculi & fistulae

TREMATODA

S. HAEMATOBIUM

S. MANSONI

The Lymphatic System

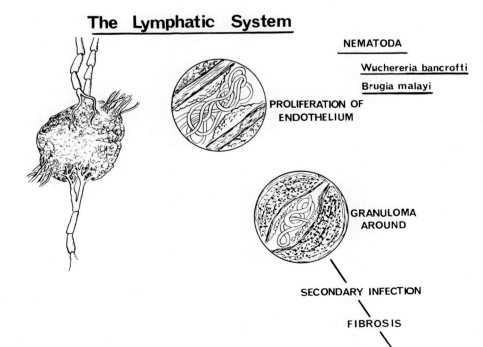

NEMATODA

Wuchereria bancrofti
Brugia malayi

PROLIFERATION OF
ENDOTHELIUM

LYMPHADENITIS
Lymphangitis
Lymph varices
ELEPHANTIASIS
Hydrocele
Chyluria, etc.

GRANULOMA
AROUND

SECONDARY INFECTION

FIBROSIS

CALCIFICATION

PLATE 120

Recapitulation (Cont)

Local effects of worm infection, continued.
The Circulatory System

TRANSIENT in blood

1. LARVAE TO PULMONARY CAPILLARIES
NEMATODA

ASCARIS   LUMBRICOIDES

STRONGYLOIDES STERCORALIS

ANCYLOSTOMA DUODENALE

Ancylostoma braziliense (human strains)

NECATOR AMERICANUS

Dirofilaria spp

Brugia malayi

Brugia pahangi

Brugia patei

   A type of visceral
   larva migrans

Haemoptysis

Pneumonia sometime

Tropical Eosinophilia

2. LARVAE TO ENCYST AT SITE OF PREDILECTION
NEMATODA

TRICHINELLA SPIRALIS

CESTODA

TAENIA SOLIUM (Cysticercus cellulosae)

ECHINOCOCCUS GRANULOSUS(Hydatid)

MULTICEPS spp.(Coenurus)

Severe constitutional symptoms in trichinosis

None per se with remainder

3. LARVAE TO MATURE TO ADULTS AT SITE OF PREDILECTION
NEMATODA

WUCHERERIA BANCROFTI

BRUGIA MALAYI

TREMATODA

Ectopic paragonimus westermani

Ectopic fasciola hepatica

None per se

4. ECTOPIC OR ANIMAL STRAIN LARVAE TO PROVOKE GRANULOMATA ANYWHERE (VISCERAL LARVA MIGRANS)

None per se

NEMATODA	CESTODA
Ascaris lumbricoides	Sparganum mansoni
Strongyloides stercoralis	Sparganum proliferum
TOXOCARA CANIS (and cati)	
Gnathostoma spinigerum	

None per se

5. ECTOPIC OVA TO PROVOKE GRANULOMATA ANYWHERE
TREMATODA

SCHISTOSOMA MANSONI	Heterophyes heterophyes
SCHISTOSOMA JAPONICUM	Metagonimus spp

None per se

MORE PERMANENT IN BLOOD

1. ADULTS LIVE IN CIRCULATORY SYSTEM

NEMATODA	TREMATODA
Sometimes Dirofilaria spp. in heart	SCHISTOSOMA HAEMATOBIUM
	SCHISTOSOMA MANSONI in veins
	SCHISTOSOMA JAPONICUM

None per se

2. LARVAE CIRCULATE   IN BLOOD
NEMATODA

WUCHERERIA BANCROFTI

BRUGIA MALAYI

LOA LOA

Dipetalonema streptocerca

Dipetalonema perstans

Mansonella ozzardi

Dirofilaria spp.

May be responsible for some general constitutional symptoms

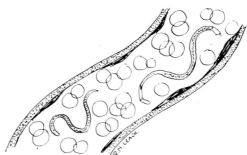

IN MYOCARDIUM LARVAE PROVOKING GRANULOMATA AND MYOCARDITIS
NEMATODA

TRICHINELLA SPIRALIS

Occasionally other ectopic larvae or ova

Myocarditis & heart failure

PLATE 121

Recapitulation (Cont.)

Local Effects of Worm Infection, continued.

Clinico–pathological correlation

The Skin and Subcutaneous Tissue

Penetration by Invading Larvae

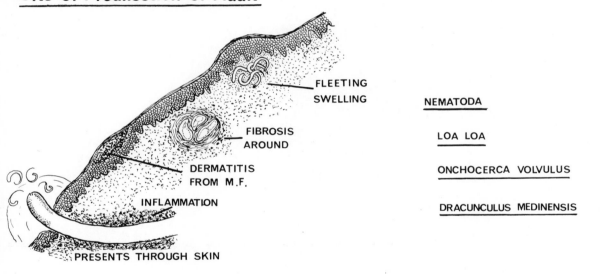

NEMATODA

TO BLOOD STREAM

STRONGYLOIDES STERCORALIS

ANCYLOSTOMA DUODENALE

A. braziliense (human strains)

NECATOR AMERICANUS

Petechial dermatitis
Swimmer's itch

ARREST IN EPIDERMIS

A·braziliense (animal strains)

A. caninum

cutaneous larva migrans

Creeping eruption

TREMATODA

SCHISTOSOMA Spp.(human strains)

SCHISTOSOMA Spp.(animal strains)

Little effect
Cercarial dermatitis

NEMATODA

FILARIAL LARVAE. Wuchereria bancrofti

Brugia malayi

None per se, or
Slight dermatitis

Site of Predilection of Adult

FLEETING SWELLING

FIBROSIS AROUND

DERMATITIS FROM M.F.

INFLAMMATION

PRESENTS THROUGH SKIN

NEMATODA

LOA LOA

ONCHOCERCA VOLVULUS

DRACUNCULUS MEDINENSIS

Calabar swelling

Fibrotic tumour
M.f. dermatitis

Ulcer

Inhabited by Ectopic Larvae

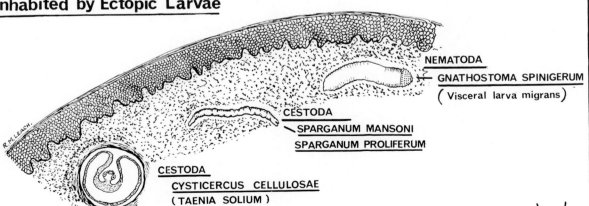

NEMATODA

GNATHOSTOMA SPINIGERUM

(Visceral larva migrans)

CESTODA

SPARGANUM MANSONI

SPARGANUM PROLIFERUM

CESTODA

CYSTICERCUS CELLULOSAE

(TAENIA SOLIUM)

Swelling
Irritation
Infection

Irritation by Adult

NEMATODA
ENTEROBIUS VERMICULARIS

Pruritis ani
and vulvae

The Muscle and Bone

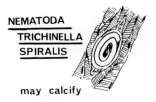

NEMATODA
TRICHINELLA SPIRALIS

may calcify

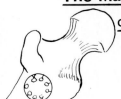

CESTODA

CYSTICERCUS CELLULOSAE (Taenia solium)

Sparganum spp.

HYDATID (Echinococcus granulosus)

Pain and swelling

Pain and spontaneous fractures